DORLAND'S
MEDICAL
ABBREVIATIONS

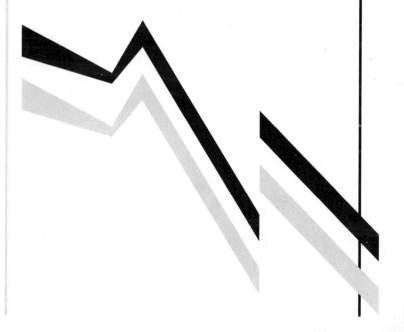

DORLAND'S
MEDICAL
ABBREVIATIONS

W. B. SAUNDERS COMPANY
Harcourt Brace Jovanovich, Inc.
Philadelphia London Toronto Montreal Sydney Tokyo

W. B. SAUNDERS COMPANY
Harcourt Brace Jovanovich, Inc.

The Curtis Center
Independence Square West
Philadelphia, PA 19106

Library of Congress Cataloging-in-Publication Data

Dorland's medical abbreviations.
       p.   cm.
     ISBN 0-7216-3751-5
     1. Medicine–Abbreviations. I. Title: Medical abbreviations.
     [DNLM: 1. Medicine–abbreviations. W 13 D7112]
R123.D66   1992
610'.148—dc20
DNLM/DLC   92-11623

Editor: Margaret M. Biblis
Designer: W. B. Saunders Staff
Cover Designer: Ellen Bodner-Zanolle
Production Manager: Carolyn Naylor
Chief Lexicographer: Douglas M. Anderson
Lexicographic Coordinator: Michelle Elliott

DORLAND'S MEDICAL ABBREVIATIONS   ISBN   0-7216-3751-5

Printed in the United States of America

Last digit is the print number: 9   8   7   6   5   4   3   2   1

Preface

The convenience afforded by the use of abbreviations in medicine has often been noted and the difficulties arising from their use deplored. Although the indiscriminate use of abbreviations can and does result in misinterpretation and confusion, the saving of time and space that they provide ensures their continued employment. The aim of *Dorland's Medical Abbreviations* is to give a comprehensive listing of abbreviations in common use.

Unfortunately for those who must decipher abbreviations, a single abbreviation may have a number of different meanings, multiple abbreviations may exist for a single term, and there are differences in usage among specialties, institutions, and regions. Because of these variations, no attempt has been made to give preference to any one meaning if a term has more than one meaning or to any one abbreviation if a term has more than one abbreviation. Abbreviations may also vary in form. They may consist of capitals or lower case letters (or combinations of the two), may or may not have periods, or may have a hyphen or a slash or no punctuation at all. As many variations as possible have been given here, with the exception of the alternate forms resulting from the use or omission of periods. For the most part, periods have been omitted, in accordance with the tendency of modern usage; they have been retained only in abbreviations for Latin terms and in a very few other instances.

Abbreviations are listed in alphabetical order. Numbers are ignored for purposes of alphabetization unless they occur in entries that are otherwise identical; an entry beginning with a number should be sought under the first letter following the number. Upper case letters precede lower case letters. Greek letters are treated as if they were Roman characters and are alphabetized following lower case letters; a table of the Greek alphabet will be found in the Appendix. The Appendix also contains abbreviations and symbols that do not fit into the alphabetical listing.

It is hoped that this book will be a useful tool for those who must deal with medical abbreviations. Because of the wide variety of abbreviations in use, however, and because of the continual inventing of new ones, it is inevitable that the user will find abbreviations and meanings that are not included in this book. We would appreciate it if you would send us any that you feel should be included but are not. Please send your additions and comments to:

Douglas M. Anderson
Chief Lexicographer
Dictionary Department
W. B. Saunders Company
The Curtis Center
Independence Square West
Philadelphia, PA 19106

Contents

A

absolute temperature
accommodation
acetum
adenine
adenosine
adult
age
akinetic
allergist
allergy
alveolar gas
ampere
amphetamine
anesthetic
anode
anterior
aqueous
area
argon
artery
atropine
auricle
axial
start of anesthesia
systemic arterial blood (as subscript)

A.

L. annum (year)
L. aqua (water)

A

absorbance
Actinomyces
activity
admittance
Anopheles
area
disintegration rate
mass number

A₁

aortic first heart sound

A₂

aortic second sound

Aₛ

standard atmosphere

Å

angstrom

Ã

cumulated activity

AII

angiotensin II

a

accommodation
arabinose
are
area
arterial blood
asymmetric
atto-
axial
total acidity

a.

L. annum (year)
L. aqua (water)
L. arteria (artery)

a

acceleration
activity (of a chemical species)
specific absorptivity

ā

L. ante (before)

α

alpha, the first letter of the Greek alphabet
Bunsen coefficient
heavy chain of IgA
optical

AA

acetic acid
achievement age
active-assistive
adenylic acid
Alcoholics Anonymous
alveolar-arterial
aminoacetone
amino acid

1

AA *(continued)*
    aminoacyl
    anticipatory avoidance
    arachidonic acid
    arteries
    ascending aorta
    atomic absorption
    Australia antigen
    automobile accident

aa.
    L. arteriae (arteries)

ĀĀ
    of each (in prescription
        writing, following the
        names of two or more
        ingredients)

A&A
    aid and attendance
    awake and aware

AAA
    abdominal aortic aneurysm
    abdominal aortic
        aneurysmectomy
    acute anxiety attack
    amalgam
    American Association of
        Anatomists
    androgenic anabolic agent

AAAA
    American Academy of
        Anesthesiologists's
        Assistants

AAAE
    amino acid–activating
        enzymes

AAALAC
    American Association for
        Accreditation in
        Laboratory Animal Care

AA-AMP
    amino acid adenylate

AAAS
    American Association for
        the Advancement of
        Science

AAATP
    Association for
        Anesthesiologist's
        Assistants Training
        Program

AAB
    American Association of
        Bioanalysts

AABB
    American Association of
        Blood Banks

AAC
    antibiotic-associated
        pseudomembranous
        colitis
    antimicrobial agents and
        chemotherapy

α_1AC
    alpha$_1$-antichymotrypsin

AACAHPO
    American Association of
        Certified Allied Health
        Personnel in
        Ophthalmology

AACC
    American Association for
        Clinical Chemistry

AACE
    American Association of
        Childbirth Education

AACIA
    American Association for
        Clinical Immunology and
        Allergy

AACN
    American Association of
        Colleges of Nursing

AACN *(continued)*
American Association of
Critical Care Nurses

AACP
American Academy of
Child Psychiatry

AACR
American Association for
Cancer Research

AAD
American Academy of
Dermatology

AADP
American Academy of
Denture Prosthetics

AADR
American Academy of
Dental Radiology

AADS
American Association of
Dental Schools

AAE
active assistance exercise
acute allergic encephalitis
American Association of
Endodontists

AAF
2-acetamidofluorene
acetic-alcohol-formalin
2-acetylaminofluorene
ascorbic acid factor

AAFP
American Academy of
Family Practice
American Association of
Family Physicians

AAG
α_1-acid glycoprotein

AAGP
American Academy of
General Practice

AAHA
American Academy of
Health Administration

AAHC
Association of Academic
Health Centers

AAHE
Association for the
Advancement of Health
Education

AAHP
American Association of
Hospital Planners

AAHPER
American Association for
Health, Physical
Education, and
Recreation

AAI
American Association of
Immunologists
atrial demand inhibited
(pacemaker code)

AAID
American Academy of
Implant Dentistry

AAIN
American Association of
Industrial Nurses

AAL
anterior axillary line

AALAS
American Association for
Laboratory Animal
Science, formerly known
as Animal Care Panel

AAM
American Academy of
Microbiology

AAMA
American Association of Medical Assistants

AAMC
American Association of Medical Colleges

AAMD
American Association on Mental Deficiency

AAME
acetylarginine methyl ester

AAMI
Association for the Advancement of Medical Instrumentation

AAMT
American Association for Medical Transcription
American Association for Music Therapy

AAN
American Academy of Neurology
American Academy of Nursing
α-amino acid nitrogen

AANA
American Association of Nurse Anesthetists

AANN
American Association of Neuroscience Nurses

AAO
American Academy of Ophthalmology
American Academy of Otolaryngology
American Association of Orthodontists
amino acid oxidase
awake, alert, and oriented

AAOHN
American Association of Occupational Health Nurses

AAOP
American Academy of Oral Pathology

AAOS
American Academy of Orthopaedic Surgeons

AAP
air at atmospheric pressure
American Academy of Pediatrics
American Academy of Pedodontics
American Academy of Periodontology
American Association of Pathologists

A-aP$_{CO_2}$
alveolar-arterial carbon dioxide

AAPA
American Academy of Physician Assistants
American Association of Pathologist Assistants

AAPB
American Association of Pathologists and Bacteriologists

AAPC
antibiotic-associated pseudomembranous colitis

AAPMR
American Academy of Physical Medicine and Rehabilitation

AAR
  antigen-antiglobulin
    reaction

AARC
  American Association for
    Respiratory Care

AAROM
  active assistive range of
    motion

AARP
  American Association of
    Retired Persons

AART
  American Association for
    Rehabilitation Therapy
  American Association of
    Respiratory Therapy

AAS
  anthrax antiserum
  aortic arch syndrome
  atomic absorption
    spectroscopy

AASH
  adrenal androgen
    stimulating hormone

AAT
  alanine aminotransferase
  α_1-antitrypsin
  atrial demand triggered
    (pacemaker code)
  auditory apperception test

AATA
  American Art Therapy
    Association

AATS
  American Association for
    Thoracic Surgery

AAV
  adeno-associated virus
  AIDS-associated virus

AB
  abnormal

AB *(continued)*
  abortion
  aid to the blind
  alcian blue
  antigen binding
  apex beat
  L. Artium Baccalaureus
    (Bachelor of Arts)
  asbestos body
  asthmatic bronchitis
  axiobuccal

A > B
  air greater than bone

A/B
  acid-base ratio

Ab
  antibody

ab
  abortion

ABA
  abscissic acid
  allergic bronchopulmonary
    aspergillosis
  American Bar Association
  American Board of
    Anesthesiology
  antibacterial activity

ABAI
  American Board of Allergy
    and Immunology

ABC
  absolute basophil count
  airway, breathing, and
    circulation
  alternative birthing center
  American Blood
    Commission
  aneurysmal bone cyst
  antigen-binding capacity
  apnea, bradycardia,
    cyanosis
  aspiration biopsy cytology
  atomic, biological, and
    chemical (warfare)
  axiobuccocervical

ABCD
doxorubicin, bleomycin, lomustine, and dacarbazine

ABCP
American Board of Cardiovascular Perfusion

ABCRS
American Board of Colon and Rectal Surgery

ABD
abdomen
abdominal
abduction
aged, blind, disabled

Abd
abdomen
abdominal

abd
abdomen
abdominal
abduct
abductor

ABDIC
doxorubicin, bleomycin sulfate, dacarbazine, lomustine, and prednisone

ABDOM
abdomen
abdominal

Abdom
abdomen
abdominal

abdom
abdomen
abdominal

abd poll
abductor pollicis

ABE
acute bacterial endocarditis

ABEM
American Board of Emergency Medicine

ABFP
American Board of Family Practice

ABG
arterial blood gases
axiobuccogingival

ABG's
arterial blood gases

ABI
ankle-brachial index
atherothrombotic brain infarction

ABIM
American Board of Internal Medicine

ABL
abetalipoproteinemia
axiobuccolingual

abl
an oncogene found in the Abelson strain of mouse leukemia virus and involved in the Philadelphia chromosome translocation in chronic granulocytic leukemia

ABLB
alternate binaural loudness balance

ABMS
Advisory Board for Medical Specialties

ABN
abnormal
abnormality

Abn
abnormal

abn
abnormal
autologous bone marrow
transplantation

ABNF
Association of Black
Nursing Faculty in
Higher Education

ABNM
American Board of
Nuclear Medicine

abnor
abnormal
abnormality

abnorm
abnormal
abnormality

ABNS
American Board of
Neurological Surgery

ABO
abortion
absent bed occupancy
American Board of
Otolaryngology
antibodies
blood group

ABOG
American Board of
Obstetrics and
Gynecology

Abor
abortion

abor
abortion

ABOS
American Board of
Orthopaedic Surgery, Inc
doxorubicin, bleomycin
sulfate, vincristine, and
streptozotocin

ABP
American Board of
Pathology
American Board of
Pediatrics
androgen-binding protein
antigen-binding protein
arterial blood pressure
doxorubicin, bleomycin,
prednisone

ABPA
allergic bronchopulmonary
aspergillosis

ABPANC
American Board of Post
Anesthesia Nursing
Certification

ABPM
ambulatory blood pressure
monitoring
American Board of
Preventive Medicine

ABPMR
American Board of
Physical Medicine and
Rehabilitation

ABP&N
American Board of
Psychiatry and
Neurology

ABPS
American Board of Plastic
Surgery

ABR
abortus-Bang ring (test)
absolute bed rest
American Board of
Radiology
auditory brain stem
response

Abr
abrasions

abr
　　abrasions

abras
　　abrasions

ABS
　　acute brain syndrome
　　alkylbenzene sulfonate
　　American Board of Surgery
　　at bedside

Abs
　　absorption

abs
　　absent
　　absolute
　　absorption

abs config
　　absolute configuration

abs. feb.
　　L. absente febre (while
　　　fever is absent)

abst
　　abstract

abstr
　　abstract

abt
　　about

ABTS
　　American Board of
　　　Thoracic Surgery
　　2,2-azine-di-(3-ethylbenzthia-
　　　zoline)-6-sulfonic acid

ABU
　　American Board of
　　　Urology

Abu
　　α-aminobutyric acid

γ-Abu
　　γ-aminobutyric acid

ABV
　　dactinomycin, bleomycin,
　　　and vincristine

ABV *(continued)*
　　doxorubicin, bleomycin,
　　　and vinblastine

ABVD
　　doxorubicin, bleomycin,
　　　vinblastine, and
　　　dacarbazine

ABW
　　actual body weight

ABX
　　antibiotics

ABY
　　acid bismuth yeast (agar)

AC
　　abdominal circumference
　　acetylcholine
　　acromioclavicular
　　adrenal cortex
　　adrenocorticoid
　　air conditioning
　　air conduction
　　all culture (broth)
　　alternating current
　　anodal closure
　　anterior chamber
　　anticoagulant
　　anticomplementary
　　anti-inflammatory
　　　corticoid
　　aortic closure
　　atriocarotid
　　auriculocarotid
　　axiocervical
　　doxorubicin and
　　　cyclophosphamide

Ac
　　acetyl
　　actinium

aC
　　symbol for
　　　arabinosylcytosine

ac
　　acute

a.c.
L. ante cibum (before meals)

@c
associated with

ACA
adenocarcinoma
American College of Angiology
American College of Apothecaries
anterior cerebral artery
anticentromere antibody
Automatic Clinical Analyzer

AC/A
accommodative convergence-accommodation ratio

acad
academy

ACAT
acyl CoA:cholesterol acyltransferase
automatic computerized axial tomography

ACB
antibody-coated bacteria

AC/BC
air conduction/bone conduction

ACC
acinic cell carcinoma
acute care center
adenoid cystic carcinomas
adrenocortical carcinoma
ambulatory care center
American College of Cardiology
anodal closure contraction
laboratory accident

Acc
acceleration
accident

Acc *(continued)*
accommodation
adenoid cystic carcinoma

acc
according

AcCh
acetylcholine

AcChR
acetylcholine receptor

AcCHS
acetylcholinesterase

accid
accident
accidental

ACCl
anodal closure clonus

AcCoA
acetylcoenzyme A

accom
accommodation

ACCP
American College of Chest Physicians

ACCR
amylase creatinine clearance ratio

accur.
L. accuratissime (most accurately)

ACD
absolute cardiac dullness
acid citrate dextrose
allergic contact dermatitis
anterior chest diameter
area of cardiac dullness

AC/DC
alternating current/direct current

ACD sol
acid citrate dextrose solution

ACE
acetonitrile
adrenocortical extract
angiotensin converting
enzyme

ACe
doxorubicin and
cyclophosphamide

Ace
acetone

ACEI
angiotensin converting
enzyme inhibitor

ACEP
American College of
Emergency Physicians

ACF
accessory clinical findings
acute care facility

ACFUCY
dactinomycin,
5-fluorouracil, and
cyclophosphamide

ACG
American College of
Gastroenterology
angiocardiography
apexcardiogram

AcG
accelerator globulin
(coagulation Factor V)

Ac-globulin
accelerator globulin

ACGME
Accreditation Council for
Graduate Medical
Education

ACH
adrenocortical hormone

ACh
acetylcholine

ACHA
American College of
Hospital Administrators

AChE
acetylcholinesterase

ACHNA
American College of
Nursing Home
Administrators

ACHNE
Association of Community
Health Nurse Education

AChR
acetylcholine receptors

AChRab
acetylcholine receptor
antibody

AC & HS
L. ante cibum et hora
somni (before meals and
at bedtime)

ACI
acoustic comfort index
adenylate cyclase inhibitor
adrenal cortical
insufficiency
anticlonus index

acid phos
acid phosphatase

acid PO$_4$
acid phosphatase

acid p'tase
acid phosphatase

ACIOC
anterior chamber
intraocular lens

ACL
anterior cruciate ligament

ACl
aspiryl chloride

ACLA
American Clinical
Laboratory Association

ACLAM
American College of
Laboratory Animal
Medicine

ACLC
Assessment of Children's
Language

ACLPS
Academy of Clinical
Laboratory Physicians
and Scientists

ACLS
advanced cardiac life
support

ACM
albumin-calcium-magnesium
doxorubicin, cyclophos-
phamide, and
methotrexate

ACN
acute conditioned necrosis

AcNeu
N-acetylneuraminic acid

AcNHFln
acetylaminofluorene

ACNM
American College of
Nuclear Medicine
American College of
Nurse-Midwives

Ac$_2$O
acetic anhydride

ACO
anodal closing odor

AcOEt
ethyl acetate

ACOG
American College of
Obstetricians and
Gynecologists

AcOH
acetic acid

ACOP
doxorubicin,
cyclophosphamide,
vincristine, and
prednisone

ACOPP
doxorubicin,
cyclophosphamide,
vincristine, procarbazine,
and prednisone

ACOS
American College of
Osteopathic Surgeons

acous
acoustic
acoustics

ACP
acid phosphatase
acyl carrier protein
American College of
Pathologists
American College of
Physicians
Animal Care Panel
anodal-closing picture
aspirin, caffeine,
phenacetin

ϵ-Acp
ϵ-aminocaproic acid

AC-PH
acid phosphatase

ACPP
adrenocorticopolypeptide

ACPS
acrocephalopolysyndactyly

ACR
>   acriflavine
>   adenomatosis of colon and
>   rectum
>   American College of
>   Radiology
>   anticonstipation regimen

Acr
>   acrylic

ACRM
>   American Congress of
>   Rehabilitation Medicine

ACS
>   acute confusional state
>   American Cancer Society
>   American College of
>   Surgeons
>   American Society of
>   Cytology
>   aperture current setting
>   Association of Clinical
>   Scientists

ACSM
>   American College of Sports
>   Medicine

ACSV
>   aortocoronary saphenous
>   vein

ACT
>   achievement through
>   counseling and treatment
>   actinomycin
>   activated clotting time
>   activated coagulation time
>   advanced coronary
>   treatment
>   anodal closure tetanus
>   anticoagulant therapy

act
>   active
>   activity

ACTA
>   American Cardiovascular
>   Technologists Association

ACTA *(continued)*
>   American Corrective
>   Therapy Association
>   Automatic Computerized
>   Transverse Axial
>   (scanner)

act-C
>   actinomycin C

act-D
>   actinomycin D

ACTe
>   anodal closure tetanus

ACTH
>   adrenocorticotropic
>   hormone

ACTH-RF
>   corticotropin
>   (adrenocorticotropic
>   hormone) releasing factor

ACTN
>   adrenocorticotropin

ACTP
>   adrenocorticotropic
>   polypeptide

ACV
>   acyclovir
>   atrial/carotid/ventricular

ACVD
>   acute cardiovascular
>   disease

ACVM
>   American College of
>   Veterinary
>   Microbiologists

ACVP
>   American College of
>   Veterinary Pathologists

AcylSCoA
>   acyl coenzyme A

AD
>   accident dispensary

AD *(continued)*
    active disease
    admitting diagnosis
    alcohol dehydrogenase
    Aleutian disease
    Alzheimer's disease
    analgesic dose
    anodal duration
    antigenic determinant
    arthritic dose
    autonomic dysreflexia
    average deviation
    axiodistal
    axis deviation

A.D.
    L. auris dextra (right ear)

A d
    anisotropic disk

A&D
    admission and discharge
    ascending and descending

ADA
    adenosine deaminase
    American Dental
        Association
    American Diabetes
        Association
    American Dietetic
        Association
    anterior descending artery

ADA #
    American Diabetes
        Association diet number

ADAA
    American Dental
        Assistants Association

ADAMHA
    Alcohol, Drug Abuse, and
        Mental Health
        Administration, an
        agency of the United
        States Public Health
        Service

ADC
    Aid to Dependent Children
    albumin, dextrose, and
        catalase (culture medium)
    analog-to-digital converter
    anodal duration
        contraction
    average daily census

ADCC
    antibody-dependent
        cell-mediated cytotoxicity

ADD
    adenosine deaminase
    attention deficit disorder
    average daily dose

add
    adding
    addition
    adduction
    adductor

add.
    L. adde (add)

ad. def. an.
    L. ad defectionem animi (to
        the point of fainting)

add poll
    adductor pollicis

ADE
    acute disseminated
        encephalitis
    apparent digestive energy

Ade
    adenine

ADEM
    acute disseminated
        encephalomyelitis

adenoca
    adenocarcinoma

ADG
    atrial diastolic gallop
    axiodistogingival

Ad grat. acid.
>   L. ad gratum aciditatem (to
>   an agreeable sourness)

ADH
>   alcohol dehydrogenase
>   antidiuretic hormone

ADHA
>   American Dental
>   Hygienists Association

Adhib.
>   L. adhibendus (to be
>   administered)

ADI
>   acceptable daily intake
>   allowable daily intake
>   axiodistoincisal

ADIC
>   doxorubicin and
>   dacarbazine

ad int.
>   L. ad interim (meanwhile)

adj
>   adjoining
>   adjunct

ADL
>   activities of daily living

ad lib.
>   L. ad libitum (at pleasure)

ADL/PDLS
>   activities of daily
>   living/daily living skills

ADM
>   administrative medicine
>   administrator

Adm
>   admission
>   admitted

adm
>   admission
>   admitted

admin
>   administer
>   administration

admov.
>   L. admove (add)
>   L. admoveatur (let there be
>   added)

ADN
>   Associate Degree in
>   Nursing

ADO
>   axiodisto-occlusal

Ado
>   adenosine

ADOAP
>   doxorubicin, vincristine,
>   cytarabine, and
>   prednisone

AdoCbl
>   adenosylcobalamin

AdoMet
>   S-adenosylmethionine

ADP
>   adenosine diphosphate
>   area diastolic pressure
>   automatic data processing

ADPase
>   adenosine diphosphatase
>   Apyrase

ADPL
>   average daily patient load

Ad pond. om.
>   L. ad pondus omnium (to
>   the weight of the whole)

ADQ
>   abductor digiti quinti M.

ADR
>   accepted dental remedies
>   adverse drug reaction
>   doxorubicin (Adriamycin)

Adr
  doxorubicin (Adriamycin)

Adria
  Adriamycin

ADS
  anatomical dead space
  antibody deficiency
    syndrome
  antidiuretic substance

ad sat.
  L. ad saturatum (to
    saturation)

adst. feb.
  L. adstante febre (while
    fever is present)

ADT
  accepted dental
    therapeutics
  adenosine triphosphate
  agar-gel diffusion test
  alternate-day therapy
  alternate-day treatment
  anodal duration tetanus
  anything desired

ADTA
  American Dance Therapy
    Association
  American Dental Trade
    Association

ADTe
  anodal duration tetanus

ad us. ext.
  L. ad usum externum (for
    external use)

ADV
  adenovirus

Adv
  advisory

adv
  advice
  advise

A-DV
  arterio-deep venous

A/DV
  arterio/deep venous

Adv.
  L. adversum (against)

advert
  advertisement
  advertising

Ad 2 vic.
  L. ad duas vices (at two
    times, for two doses)

A5D5W
  alcohol 5 per cent, dextrose
    5 per cent in water

ADX
  adrenalectomized

AE
  above elbow
  acrodermatitis
    enteropathica
  anoxic encephalopathy
  antitoxineinheit (antitoxin
    unit)
  apoenzyme
  aryepiglottic
  energy of activation

A-E
  above the elbow
    (amputation)

A + E
  analysis and evaluation

ae.
  L. aetatis (of the age)

AEA
  alcohol, ether, acetone

AEC
  at earliest convenience
  Atomic Energy
    Commission

AEG
   air encephalogram

Aeg.
   L. aeger, aegra (the
      patient)

AEM
   analytical electron
      microscope
   analytical electron
      microscopy

AEP
   artificial endocrine
      pancreas
   auditory evoked potential
   average evoked potential

AEq
   age equivalent

AER
   acoustic evoked potential
   aldosterone excretion rate
   auditory evoked response
   average evoked response

Aero
   Aerobacter

AES
   American
      Electroencephalographic
      Society

AET
   absorption-equivalent
      thickness

aet.
   L. aetas (age)

aetat.
   L. aetatis (of the age)

AF
   abnormal frequency
   acid-fast
   aflatoxin
   albumose-free
   aldehyde fuchsin
   amniotic fluid
   angiogenesis factor

AF *(continued)*
   antibody-forming
   aortic flow
   atrial fibrillation
   atrial flutter

A-F
   antifibrinogen

af
   audio-frequency

AFB
   acid-fast bacillus
   acid-fast bacteria
   aflatoxin B

AFBG
   aortofemoral bypass graft

AFC
   antibody-forming cells

AFCR
   American Federation for
      Clinical Research

AFDC
   Aid to Families with
      Dependent Children

afeb
   afebrile

aff
   afferent

AFG
   aflatoxin G
   amniotic fluid glucose

AFH
   anterior facial height

AFI
   amaurotic familial idiocy

AFib
   atrial fibrillation

A fib
   atrial fibrillation

AFID
   alkali flame ionization
      detectors

AFIP
Armed Forces Institute of
Pathology

AFL
aflatoxicol
anti–fatty liver
atrial flutter

AFl
atrial flutter

AFM
aflatoxin M

AFO
ankle-foot orthosis

AFP
alpha-fetoprotein
anterior faucial pillar

AFPP
acute fibrinopurulent
pneumonia

AFQ
aflatoxin Q

AFQT
Armed Forces
Qualification Test

AFR
ascorbic free radical

AFRD
acute febrile respiratory
disease

AFRI
acute febrile respiratory
illness

AFS
American Fertility Society

AFSP
acute fibrinoserous
pneumonia

AFT
aflatoxin

AFTC
apparently free
testosterone
concentration

AFTN
autonomously functioning
thyroid nodule

AFV
amniotic fluid volume

AG
analytical grade
antiglobulin
antigravity
atrial gallop
axiogingival

A/G
albumin-globulin ratio

Ag
antigen
silver

AGA
accelerated growth area
American
Gastroenterological
Association
appropriate for gestational
age

Ag-Ab
antigen-antibody (complex)

AGCT
Army General
Classification Test

AGD
agarose diffusion (method)

AGE
acute gastroenteritis
agarose gel electrophoresis
angle of greatest extension

AGEPC
acetyl glyceryl ether
phosphoryl choline

AGF
> angle of greatest flexion

AGG
> agammaglobulinemia

agg
> agglutinate
> agglutination
> aggregate

aggl
> agglutinate
> agglutination

aggred. feb.
> L. aggrediente febre (while the fever is coming on)

AGGS
> anti–gas gangrene serum

AgI
> silver iodide

agit
> L. agita (shake)

agit. a. us.
> L. agita ante usum (shake before using)

agit. bene
> L. agita bene (shake well)

Agit. vas.
> L. agitato vase (the vial being shaken)

AGL
> acute granulocytic leukemia
> aminoglutethimide

AGMK
> African green monkey kidney (tissue culture)

AGN
> acute glomerulonephritis
> agnosia

AgNO₃
> silver nitrate

AGP
> acid glycoprotein
> agar-gel precipitation

AGPT
> agar-gel precipitation test

A/G ratio
> albumin/globulin ratio

AGS
> adrenogenital syndrome
> American Geriatrics Society

AGT
> antiglobulin test

agt
> agent

AGTH
> adrenoglomerulotropin

AGTT
> abnormal glucose tolerance test

AGV
> aniline gentian violet

AH
> abdominal hysterectomy
> accidental hypothermia
> acetohexamide
> afterhyperpolarization
> amenorrhea and hirsutism
> aminohippurate
> anterior hypothalamus
> antihyaluronidase
> arterial hypertension
> artificial heart
> ascites hepatoma
> autonomic hyperreflexia

A&H
> accident and health insurance

A h
> ampere-hour

ah
   hyperopic astigmatism

AHA
   acetohydroxamic acid
   acquired hemolytic anemia
   American Heart
      Association
   American Hospital
      Association
   anterior hypothalamic
      area
   aspartylhydroxamic acid
   autoimmune hemolytic
      anemia

AHC
   acute hemorrhagic
      conjunctivitis
   acute hemorrhagic cystitis

AHCPR
   Agency for Health Care
      Policy and Research

AHD
   arteriosclerotic heart
      disease
   atherosclerotic heart
      disease
   autoimmune hemolytic
      disease

AHE
   acute hemorrhagic
      encephalomyelitis

AHES
   artificial heart energy
      system

AHF
   acute heart failure
   American Hospital
      Formulary
   antihemolytic factor
   antihemophilic factor

AHG
   aggregated human globulin
   antihemophilic globulin
   antihuman globulin

AHGS
   acute herpetic gingival
      stomatitis

AHH
   alpha-hydrazine analog of
      histidine
   arylhydrocarbon
      hydroxylase

AHI
   active hostility index

AHLE
   acute hemorrhagic
      leukoencephalitis

AHLS
   antihuman lymphocyte
      serum

AHM
   ambulatory Holter
      monitoring

AHMI
   American Holistic Medical
      Institute

AHP
   acute hemorrhagic
      pancreatitis
   air at high pressure
   Assistant House Physician

AHPA
   American Health Planning
      Association

AHPAT
   Allied Health Practitioners
      Aptitude/Admission test

AHS
   Assistant House Surgeon

AHT
   antihyaluronidase titer
   augmented histamine test

AHTG
   antihuman thymocyte
      globulin

AHuG
   aggregated human IgG

AI
   accidentally incurred
   anaphylatoxin inhibitor
   aortic incompetence
   aortic insufficiency
   apical impulse
   artificial insemination
   artificial intelligence
   axioincisal

A&I
   Allergy and Immunology
   (Service)

AIA
   allylisopropylacetamide
   amylase inhibitor activity

AIBA
   aminoisobutyric acid

AIBS
   American Institute of
   Biological Sciences

AIC
   aminoimidazole
   carboxamide
   Association des Infirmières
   Canadiennes

AICA
   anterior inferior cerebellar
   artery
   anterior inferior
   communicating artery

AICD
   automatic implantable
   cardioverter-defibrillator

AICF
   autoimmune complement
   fixation

AID
   acute infectious disease
   artificial insemination by
   donor (heterologous
   insemination)

AID *(continued)*
   artificial insemination
   donor
   autoimmune deficiency
   autoimmune disease

AIDS
   acquired immunodeficiency
   syndrome

AIE
   acute infectious
   encephalitis

AIEP
   amount of insulin
   extractable from the
   pancreas

AIH
   American Institute of
   Homeopathy
   artificial insemination by
   husband (homologous
   insemination)

AIHA
   American Industrial
   Hygiene Association
   autoimmune hemolytic
   anemia

AIL
   angioimmunoblastic
   lymphadenopathy

AILD
   angioimmunoblastic
   lymphadenopathy with
   dysproteinemia

AIM
   acute intermittent
   porphyria
   Artificial Intelligence in
   Medicine

AIMS
   abnormal involuntary
   movement scale

AIN
   acute interstitial nephritis

AINS
    anti-inflammatory
      nonsteroidal

AIO
    amyloid of
      immunoglobulin origin

AIP
    acute intermittent
      porphyria
    automated
      immunoprecipitation
    average intravascular
      pressure

AIR
    aminoimidazole
      ribonucleotide

AIS
    abbreviated injury score
    androgen insensitivity
      syndrome
    anti-insulin serum

AITT
    arginine insulin tolerance
      test

AIU
    absolute iodine uptake

AIUM
    American Institute of
      Ultrasound in Medicine

AIVR
    accelerated idioventricular
      rhythm

AJ
    ankle jerk

AJCC
    American Joint Committee
      on Cancer

AJCCS
    American Joint Committee
      on Cancer Staging

AK
    above knee

AK *(continued)*
    adenylate kinase

A-K
    above the knee

AKA
    above-knee amputation
    alcoholic ketoacidosis
    also known as

a.k.a.
    also known as

AK amp
    above-knee amputation

AL
    acute leukemia
    adaptation level
    albumin
    alignment mark
    auris laeva
    axiolingual

Al
    aluminum

ALA
    δ-aminolevulinic acid
    axiolabial

Ala
    alanine
    alanyl

AlaAT
    alanine aminotransferase

ALAD
    abnormal left axis
      deviation
    aminolevulinic acid
      dehydrase

ALAG
    axiolabiogingival

ALAL
    axiolabiolingual

ALAT
    alanine aminotransferase
    alanine transaminase

alb
  albumin

ALC
  approximate lethal
    concentration
  avian leukosis complex
  axiolinguocervical

alc
  alcohol
  alcoholic
  ethanol
  ethyl alcohol

alcoh
  alcohol
  alcoholic
  ethanol
  ethyl alcohol

ALD
  adrenoleukodystrophy
  alcoholic liver disease
  aldolase

ALG
  antilymphocyte globulin
  axiolinguogingival

ALGOL
  algorithmic oriented
    language

ALH
  anterior lobe hormone
  anterior lobe of the
    hypophysis

alk
  alkaline

Alk phos
  alkaline phosphatase

alk phos
  alkaline phosphatase

Alk PO$_4$ tase
  alkaline phosphatase

alk p'tase
  alkaline phosphatase

ALL
  acute lymphatic leukemia
  acute lymphoblastic
    leukemia
  acute lymphocytic
    leukemia
  allergies
  allergy

All
  allose

ALM
  acral lentiginous
    melanoma
  alveolar lining material

ALME
  acetyl-lysine methyl ester

ALMI
  anterolateral myocardial
    infarction

ALN
  anterior lymph node

ALO
  axiolinguo-occlusal

ALOMAD
  doxorubicin, chlorambucil,
    vincristine

ALOS
  average length of stay

ALP
  alkaline phosphatase
  anterior lobe of pituitary
  antilymphocyte plasma

ALRR
  arthroscopic lateral
    retinacular release

ALPS
  Aphasia Languages
    Performance Scales

ALS
  acute lateral sclerosis
  advanced life support

ALS *(continued)*
    amyotrophic lateral
        sclerosis
    angiotensin-like substance
    anterolateral sclerosis
    anticipated life span
    antilymphatic serum
    antilymphocyte serum

ALT
    alanine aminotransferase
    alanine transaminase
    alternate
    altitude
    argon laser trabeculoplasty

ALT/AST ratio
    alanine aminotransferase
        to aspartate

ALTB
    acute
        laryngotracheobronchitis

Alt. dieb.
    L. alternis diebus (every
        other day)

ALTEE
    acetyl-L-tyrosine ethyl
        ester

Alt. hor.
    L. alternis horis (every
        other hour)

Alt. noc.
    L. alterna nocte (every
        other night)

ALU
    arithmetic and logic unit

ALV
    alveolar
    avian leukosis virus

alv
    alveolar

alv. adst.
    L. alvo adstricta (when the
        bowels are constipated)

ALW
    arch-loop-whorl system

AM
    actomyosin
    aerospace medicine
    alveolar macrophage
    ametropia
    amperemeter
    ampicillin
    amplitude modulation
    anovular menstruation
    antibodies to cardiac
        myosin
    arithmetic mean
    arousal mechanism
    L. Artium Magister
        (Master of Arts)
    aviation medicine
    axiomesial
    myopic astigmatism

Am
    americium

am
    ametropia
    meter angle
    myopic astigmatism

a.m.
    L. ante meridiem (before
        noon)

a2M
    alpha-2 macroglobulin

AMA
    Aerospace Medical
        Association
    American Medical
        Association
    antimitochondrial antibody

AMA-ERF
    AMA Education &
        Research Foundation

AMAL
    Aero-Medical Acceleration
        Laboratory

AMAP
as much as possible

AMAT
amorphous material

A-MAT
amorphous material

amb
ambulance
ambulate
ambulatory

ambig
ambiguous

AMC
antimalaria campaign
arm muscle circumference
arthrogryposis multiplex
congenita
axiomesiocervical

AMD
aeromedical data
alpha-methyldopa
arthroscopic
microdiskectomy
axiomesiodistal

AMEA
American Medical
Electroencephalographic
Association

AMegL
acute megokaryoblastic
leukemia

Amer
American

AMF
antimuscle factor

Amf
amniotic fluid

AMG
alpha$_2$-macroglobulin
antimacrophage globulin
axiomesiogingival

Amh
mixed astigmatism with
myopia predominating

AMI
acute myocardial
infarction
amitriptyline
anterior myocardial
infarction
Association of Medical
Illustrators
axiomesioincisal

AML
acute monocytic leukemia
acute myeloblastic
leukemia
acute myelocytic leukemia
acute myelogenous
leukemia
acute myeloid leukemia
anterior mitral leaflet

AMLR
autologous mixed
lymphocyte reaction

AMLS
antimouse lymphocyte
serum

AMM
agnogenic myeloid
metaplasia
ammonia

AMML
acute myelomonocytic
leukemia

AMMOL
acute myelomonoblastic
leukemia
acute myelomonoblastic
lymphoma

AMN
alloxazine mononucleotide

AMO
axiomesio-occlusal

AMOL
    acute monoblastic
        leukemia
    acute monocytic leukemia

amorph
    amorphous

AMP
    acid mucopolysaccharide
    adenosine monophosphate
    2-amino-2-methyl-1-propan-
        ol
    amphetamine
    ampicillin
    ampule
    amputation
    average mean pressure

3′, 5′-AMP
    cyclic adenosine
        monophosphate

amp
    amperage
    ampere
    amplification
    ampule
    amputated

AMPase
    adenosine
        monophosphatase

AMPH
    amphetamine

amph
    amphoric

amp-hr
    ampere-hour

ampl.
    L. amplus (large)

AMPS
    abnormal
        mucopolysacchariduria
    acid mucopolysaccharides

AMRA
    American Medical Record
        Association

AMRL
    Aerospace Medical
        Research Laboratories

AMS
    acute mountain sickness
    aggravated in military
        service
    American Meteorological
        Society
    amylase
    antimacrophage serum
    Army Medical Service
        (British)
    atypical measles syndrome
    auditory memory span
    automated multiphasic
        screening

ams.
    amount of a substance

AMSA
    American Medical Student
        Association
    amsacrine

Amsa
    amsacrine

AmSECT
    American Society of
        Extra-Corporeal
        Technology

AMT
    alpha-methyltyrosine
    American Medical
        Technologists
    amethopterin
    amphetamine

amt
    amount

am't
    amount

amu
    atomic mass unit

AMV
assisted mechanical
ventilation

AMWA
American Medical
Women's Association
American Medical Writers'
Association

AMX
amoxicillin

AMY
amylase

AMZ
anteromedial displacement
osteotomy

AN
anorexia nervosa
antenatal
aneurysm
aseptic necrosis
avascular necrosis

A/N
as needed

An
anisometropia
anodal
anode

ANA
American Nurses'
Association
anesthesia
anesthetic
antinuclear antibodies
aspartyl naphthylamide

ANAD
anorexia nervosa and
associated disorders

anal
analgesia
analgesic
analyses

ANAP
agglutination negative,
absorption positive

anat.
anatomical
anatomy

ANC
absolute neutrophil count

AnCC
anodal closure contraction

ANCOVA
analysis of covariance

ANDA
abbreviated new drug
application

ANDRO
androsterone

AnDTe
anodal duration tetanus

anes
anesthesia
anesthetic

anesth
anesthesia
anesthetic

an ex
anode excitation

ANF
alpha-naphthoflavone
American Nurses
Foundation
antinuclear factor
atrial natriuretic factor

ang
angiogram
angle

angio
angiography

anh
anhydrous

anhydr
anhydrous

ANISO
anisocytosis

Anisometr
anisometropia

ANIT
alpha-naphthylisothicy-
anate

ank
ankle

ANLL
acute nonlymphoblastic
leukemia
acute nonlymphocytic
leukemia

Ann
annals
annual

Annls
annals

AnOC
anodal opening contraction

ANOVA
analysis of variance

ANP
A-norprogesterone

ANRC
American National Red
Cross

ANS
anterior nasal spine
antineutrophilic serum
arteriolonephrosclerosis
autonomic nervous system

ans
answer

ANSA
aminonaphtholsulfonic
acid

ANSI
American National
Standards Institute

ANT
acoustic noise test

ant.
anterior

Ant A
antamycin A

antag
antagonistic

ant al line
anterior axillary line

Anthrop
anthropology

anti-coag
anticoagulant

anti-DNA
anti-deoxyribonucleic acid

anti-GBM
antiglomerular basement
membrane

anti-HAA
antibody to hepatitis-
associated antigen

anti-HB$_S$Ag
antibody to hepatitis B
surface antigen

anti–HLTD III
antibody screen in testing
for AIDS

anti-log
antilogarithm

anti-S
anti–sulfanilic acid

Ant pit
anterior pituitary

ant pit
anterior pituitary

ANTR
apparent net transfer rate

ant sup sp
anterior superior spine

ant sup spine
anterior superior spine

ANTU
alpha-naphthylthiourea

ANUG
acute necrotizing
ulcerative gingivitis

anx
anxiety

AO
acid output
acridine orange
anodal opening
anterior oblique
aorta
aortic opening
atomic orbital
axio-occlusal
opening of the
atrioventricular valves

A-O
acoustic-optic

A/O
alert and oriented

Ao
aorta

AOA
Alpha Omega Alpha, an
honorary medical society
American Optometric
Association
American Orthopsychiatric
Association
American Osteopathic
Association

AOAA
aminooxyacetic acid

AOB
accessory olfactory bulb
alcohol on breath

AOC
abridged ocular chart
anodal opening contraction

AOCl
anodal opening clonus

AOD
arterial occlusive disease
auriculo-osteodysplasia

AODM
adult onset diabetes
mellitus

AOL
acro-osteolysis

AOM
acute otitis media

AOMA
American Occupational
Medical Association

AONE
American Organization of
Nurse Executives

AOO
anodal opening odor
atrial asynchronous
(pacemaker code)

AOP
anodal opening picture
aortic pressure
Association of Operating
Room Nurses

AoP
left ventricle to aorta
pressure gradient

aort regurg
aortic regurgitation

aort sten
aortic stenosis

AOS

anodal opening sound

AOTA

American Occupational
Therapy Association

AOTe

anodal opening tetanus

AOU

apparent oxygen
utilization

AP

acid phosphatase
action potential
acute proliferative
alkaline phosphatase
aminopeptidase
angina pectoris
antepartum
anterior pituitary (gland)
anteroposterior
aortic pressure
apical pulse
apothecary
appendectomy
appendix
arithmetic progression
arterial pressure
artificial pneumothorax
association period
atrial pacing
atrium pace
axiopulpal

A-P

anterior-posterior

A/P

ascites-plasma ratio

A&P

anterior and posterior
assessment and plan
auscultation and palpation
auscultation and
percussion

$A_2 < P_2$

aortic second sound less
than pulmonary second
sound

$A_2 > P_2$

aortic second sound greater
than pulmonary second
sound

3-AP

3-acetylpyridine

a.p.

L. ante prandium (before
dinner)

a&p

abdominal and perineal

APA

aldosterone-producing
adenoma
American Pharmaceutical
Association
American Podiatric
Association
American Psychiatric
Association
American Psychological
Association
aminopenicillanic acid
antipernicious anemia
factor

6-APA

6-aminopenicillanic acid

APACHE

Acute Physiology and
Chronic Health
Evaluation

APAF

antipernicious anemia
factor

APAP

Association of Physician
Assistants Programs

APB

    abductor pollicis brevis
    atrial premature beat

APC

    acetylsalicylic acid, phenacetin, and caffeine
    adenoidal-pharyngeal-conjunctival
    amsacrine, prednisone, and chlorambucil
    antigen-presenting cell
    antiphlogistic corticoid
    aperture current
    apneustic center
    atrial premature complex
    atrial premature contraction

APC-C

    aspirin, phenacetin, and caffeine with codeine

APCD

    adult polycystic kidney disease

APCF

    acute pharyngoconjunctival fever

APCG

    apexcardiogram

APD

    action-potential duration
    afferent pupillary defect
    anteroposterior diameter
    atrial premature depolarization

A-PD

    anteroposterior diameter

APE

    acetone powder extract
    aminophylline, phenobarbital, and ephedrine

APE *(continued)*

    anterior pituitary extract

APF

    acidulated phosphofluoride
    anabolism-promoting factor
    animal protein factor

APG

    acid-precipitable globulin

APGAR

    adaptability, partnership, growth, affection, resolve

APGL

    alkaline phosphatase activity of the granular leukocytes

APH

    adenohypophyseal hormone
    antepartum hemorrhage
    anterior pituitary hormone

APHA

    American Public Health Association

APhA

    American Pharmaceutical Association

APHP

    anti-*Pseudomonas* human plasma

$\alpha_1 PI$

    human α_1 proteinase inhibitor

APIC

    Association of Practitioners in Infection Control

APIM

    Association Professionnelle Internationale des Médecins

APKD
>adult polycystic kidney
>   disease
>adult-onset polycystic
>   kidney disease

APL
>abductor pollicis longus
>accelerated painless labor
>acute promyelocytic
>   leukemia
>anterior pituitary-like
>   (hormone)
>trademark for a brand of
>   chorionic gonadotropin

AP & Lat
>anteroposterior and lateral

A-P & Lat
>anterior-posterior and
>   lateral

APLD
>automated percutaneous
>   microdiskectomy

APM
>acid precipitable material
>anterior papillary muscle

APN
>acute pyelonephritis
>average peak noise

APO
>apomorphine
>doxorubicin, prednisone,
>   vincristine,
>   6-mercaptopurine,
>   asparaginase, and
>   methotrexate

Apo C
>apolipoprotein C

Apo D
>apolipoprotein D

Apo E
>apolipoprotein E

apoth
>apothecary

APP
>alum-precipitated protein
>alum-precipitated pyridine
>appendix

app
>apparent
>appendix

appar
>apparatus
>apparent

appl
>appliance
>application
>applied

applan
>L. applanatus (flat)

applicand
>L. applicandus (to be
>   administered)

appoint
>appointment

appr
>approximate
>approximately

approx
>approximate
>approximately

appt
>appointment

appy
>appendectomy

Appx
>appendix

APR
>abdominal-perineal
>   resection
>acute phase reactant
>amebic prevalence rate
>anterior pituitary reaction

aprax
>apraxia

APRT
adenine phosphoribosyl transferase

APS
Acute Pain Services
adenosine phosphosulfate
American Physiological Society

APT
alum-precipitated toxoid

APTA
American Physical Therapy Association

APTD
ambient temperature and pressure dry

APTT
activated partial thromboplastin time

aPTT
activated partial thromboplastin time

APUD
amine precursor uptake and decarboxylation

AQ
accomplishment quotient
achievement quotient
any quantity

Aq.
L. aqua (water)

aq
aqueous

Aq. bull.
L. aqua bulliens (boiling water)

Aq. dest.
L. aqua destillata (distilled water)

Aq. ferv.
L. aqua fervens (hot water)

Aq. frig.
L. aqua frigida (cold water)

Aq. pur.
L. aqua pura (pure water)

AQRS
in electrocardiography, the symbol for the mean manifest electrical axis of the QRS complex, measured in degrees and microvolt seconds

Aq. tep.
L. aqua tepida (tepid water)

AR
achievement ratio
active resistance
alarm reaction
allergic rhinitis
analytical reagent
androgen receptor
aortic regurgitation
Argyll Robertson (pupil)
articulare
artificial respiration
at risk
autoradiography

A/R
apical/radial

A&R
advised and released

Ar
argon
aryl group

Ara
arabinose

ara-A
adenine arabinoside

ara-C
cytarabine
cytosine arabinoside

ARAD
> abnormal right axis deviation

ARB
> any reliable brand

ARBOR
> arthropod-borne virus

ARC
> accelerating rate calorimeter
> AIDS-related complex
> American Red Cross
> anomalous retinal correspondence
> arcuate nucleus

ARCA
> acquired red cell aplasia
> American Rehabilitation Counseling Association

ArCO
> aromatic acyl radical

ARD
> absolute reaction of degeneration
> acute respiratory disease
> adult respiratory disease
> anorectal dressing
> arthritis and rheumatic diseases

ARDS
> acute respiratory distress syndrome
> adult respiratory distress syndrome

ARF
> acute renal failure
> acute respiratory failure
> acute rheumatic fever

Arg
> arginine
> arginyl

arg.
> L. argentum (silver)

ARI
> airway reactivity index

ARIA
> automated radioimmunoassay

ARL
> average remaining lifetime

ARM
> allergy relief medicine
> artificial rupture of membranes
> atomic resolution microscope

Arm
> arm amputation

ARMD
> age-related macular degeneration

ARN
> Association of Rehabilitation Nurses

AROA
> autosomal recessive ocular albinism

AROM
> active range of motion
> artificial rupture of membranes

ARP
> absolute refractory period
> Advanced Research Projects
> at-risk period

ARROM
> active resistive range of motion

ARRS
> American Roentgen Ray Society

ARRT
American Registry of
Radiologic Technologists

ARS
alizarin red S
antirabies serum

ARSM
acute respiratory system
malfunction

ART
absolute retention time
Accredited Record
Technician
Achilles tendon reflex test
acoustic reflex test
artery
automated reagin test

art
arterial
artery
articulation
artificial

arthr
arthrotomy

artic
articulation

artif
artificial

art insem
artificial insemination

ARV
AIDS-related virus
anterior right ventricular

ARVO
Association for Research in
Vision and
Ophthalmology

AS
acetylstrophanthidin
Adams-Stokes (disease)
alveolar sac
androsterone sulfate

AS *(continued)*
ankylosing spondylitis
antistreptolysin
anxiety state
aortic stenosis
arteriosclerosis
artificial sweetener
atherosclerosis
audiogenic seizure

A.S.
L. auris sinistra (left ear)

As
arsenic

As.
astigmatism

A-s
ampere-second

ASA
acetylsalicylic acid
Adams-Stokes attack
American Society of
Anesthesiologists
American Standards
Association
American Surgical
Association
argininosuccinic acid
arylsulfatase-A

Asa
β-carboxyaspartic acid

ASAHP
American Society of Allied
Health Professionals

ASAI
aortic stenosis and aortic
insufficiency

ASAP
as soon as possible

ASAS
American Society of
Abdominal Surgeons
argininosuccinic acid
synthetase

ASAT

aspartate
aminotransferase

ASB

American Society of
Bacteriologists

ASC

altered state of
consciousness
ambulatory surgical center
American Society of
Cytotechnology
ascorbic acid

ASCAD

arteriosclerotic coronary
artery disease

ASCH

American Society of
Clinical Hypnosis

ASCI

American Society for
Clinical Investigation

ASCII

American Standard Code
for Information
Interchange

Ascit Fl

ascitic fluid

ASCLT

American Society of
Clinical Laboratory
Technicians

ASCO

American Society of
Clinical Oncology
American Society of
Contemporary
Ophthalmology

ASCP

American Society of
Clinical Pathologists

ASCVD

arteriosclerotic
cardiovascular disease
atherosclerotic
cardiovascular disease

ASD

aldosterone secretion
defect
atrial septal defect

ASDC

American Society of
Dentistry for Children

ASDH

acute subdural hematoma

ASE

American Society of
Echocardiography
axilla, shoulder, elbow

ASEP

American Society for
Experimental Pathology

ASES

American shoulder and
elbow system

ASET

American Society of
Electroencephalographic
Technologists

ASF

aniline, sulfur, and
formaldehyde

ASGE

American Society of
Gastrointestinal
Endoscopy

ASH

American Society for
Hematology
asymmetrical septal
hypertrophy

AsH
> hypermetropic astigmatism
> hyperopic astigmatism

ASHA
> American School Health Association
> American Speech and Hearing Association

ASHD
> arteriosclerotic heart disease
> atherosclerotic heart disease

ASHN
> acute sclerosing hyaline necrosis

ASHP
> American Society of Hospital Pharmacists

ASIF
> Association for the Study of Internal Fixation

ASII
> American Science Information Institute

ASIM
> American Society of Internal Medicine

ASIS
> anterior superior iliac spine
> anterosuperior iliac spine

ASK
> antistreptokinase

ASL
> antistreptolysin
> argininosuccinate lyase

ASLO
> antistreptolysin-O

ASM
> American Society for Microbiology
> myopic astigmatism

ASMA
> antismooth muscle antibody

ASMI
> anteroseptal myocardial infarct

ASMR
> age-standardized mortality ratio

ASMRO
> Armed Services Medical Regulating Office

ASMT
> American Society for Medical Technology

ASN
> alkali-soluble nitrogen

ASMA

Asn
> asparagine
> asparaginyl

ASNSA
> American Society of Nursing Service Administrators

ASO
> allele-specific oligonucleotide
> antistreptolysin O
> arteriosclerosis obliterans

ASP
> American Society of Parasitologists
> area systolic pressure
> L-asparaginase

Asp
> L-asparaginase

Asp *(continued)*
    aspartic acid
    aspartyl

ASPAN
    American Society of Post
    Anesthesia Nurses

AspAT
    aspartate
    aminotransferase
    aspartate transaminase

ASPET
    American Society for
    Pharmacology and
    Experimental
    Therapeutics

ASPH
    Association of Schools of
    Public Health

ASPVD
    arteriosclerotic peripheral
    vascular disease

ASR
    aldosterone secretion rate
    aldosterone secretory rate

ASRT
    American Society of
    Radiologic Technologists

ASS
    anterior superior spine
    argininosuccinate
    synthetase

assoc
    associate
    associated
    association

asst
    adult situational stress
    reaction
    assistant

AST
    angiotensin sensitivity test
    aspartate
    aminotransferase

AST *(continued)*
    aspartate transaminase
    Association of Surgical
    Technologists

Ast.
    astigmatism

ASTDN
    Association of State and
    Territorial Directors of
    Nursing

Asth.
    asthenopia

ASTI
    antispasticity index

Astigm
    astigmatism

ASTM
    American Society for
    Testing and Materials

ASTO
    antistreptolysin-O

as tol
    as tolerated

ASTR
    American Society for
    Therapeutic Radiology

ASTZ
    antistreptozyme

ASUTS
    American Society of
    Ultrasound Technical
    Specialists

ASV
    anodic stripping
    voltammetry
    antisnake venom
    arterio–superficial venous

A-SV
    arterio–superficial venous

A/SV
    arterio–superficial venous

ASVG

autologous saphenous vein
graft

ASX

asymptomatic

Asx

asparaginyl
aspartyl
symbol meaning "Asp or
Asn"

asym

asymmetrical

AT

achievement test
Achilles tendon
adenine and thymine
adjunctive therapy
air temperature
Ger. alt Tuberculin (Old
Tuberculin)
aminotransferase
amitriptyline
anaphylotoxin
antithrombin
antitrypsin
applanation tonometry
atrial tachycardia
attenuated
attenuation

AT$_{10}$

dihydrotachysterol

AT-III

antithrombin III

At

astatine
in electrocardiography,
symbol for the mean
manifest direction and
magnitude of
repolarization of the
myocardium determined
algebraically and
measured in degrees and
microvolt seconds

at

atomic

ATA

alimentary toxic aleukia
antithyroglobulin antibody
anti-*Toxoplasma*
antibodies
atmosphere absolute
aurintricarboxylic acid

ATC

activated thymus cell
around the clock

ATCC

American Type Culture
Collection

ATD

Alzheimer-type dementia
anthropomorphic test
dummy
antithyroid drugs
asphyxiating thoracic
dystrophy

ATE

adipose tissue extract

ATEE

acetyltyrosine ethyl ester

At Fib

atrial fibrillation

at fib

atrial fibrillation

ATG

adenine, thymine, and
guanine
antihuman thymocyte
globulin
antithymocyte globulin
antithyroglobulin

ATGAM

antithymocyte gamma
globulin

ATHC

3α-allotetrahydrocortisol

Athsc
atherosclerosis

ATL
Achilles tendon
lengthening
adult T-cell
leukemia/lymphoma
antitension line
atypical lymphocytes

ATLA
adult T-cell leukemia
antigen

ATLS
advanced trauma life
support

ATLV
adult T-cell leukemia virus

atm
atmosphere
atmospheric
standard atmosphere

ATN
tyrosinase-negative (ty-neg)
oculocutaneous albinism

ATNC
atraumatic, normocephalic

at. no.
atomic number

ATNR
asymmetric tonic neck
reflex

ATP
adenosine triphosphate

ATPase
adenosine triphosphatase

ATPD
symbol indicating that a
gas volume has been
expressed as if it had been
dried at the ambient
temperature and pressure

ATPS
ambient temperature and
pressure, saturated

ATR
Achilles tendon reflex

atr
atrophy

atr fib
atrial fibrillation

ATS
American Thoracic Society
antitetanic serum
antithymocyte serum
anxiety tension state
arteriosclerosis

ATSDR
Agency for Toxic
Substances and Diseases
Registry, an agency of the
United States Public
Health Service

ATT
arginine tolerance test

at vol
atomic volume

At wt
atomic weight

ATZ
atypical transformation
zone

AU
Ångström unit
antitoxin unit
arbitrary units
L. aures unitas (both ears
together)
L. auris uterque (each ear)
azauridine

Au
gold (L. aurum)
Australian antigen

^{198}Au
  radioactive gold

Au(1)
  Australia antigen

AUA
  American Urological
  Association

Au Ag
  Australia antigen

AuAg
  Australia antigen

AuBMT
  autologous bone marrow
  transplantation

auct.
  L. auctorum (of authors)

aud
  auditory

AUG
  acute ulcerative gingivitis

AUHAA
  Australia
  hepatitis-associated
  antigen

AUL
  acute undifferentiated
  leukemia

AUO
  amyloid of unknown origin

AUPHA
  Association of University
  Programs in Health
  Administration

aur
  L. auris (ear)

aur.
  L. aurum (gold)

aur fib
  auricular fibrillation

auric.
  auricular

aus
  auscultation

ausc
  auscultation

AuSH
  Australia serum hepatitis

AuSh
  Australia serum hepatitis

AUTS
  Adult Use of Tobacco
  Survey

aux
  auxiliary

AV
  alveolar duct
  anterior-ventral
  anteversion
  anteverted
  antivirin
  aortic valve
  arteriovenous
  atrioventricular
  auriculoventricular node
  doxorubicin and vincristine

Av
  average
  avoirdupois

aV
  augmented unipolar limb
  lead

AVA
  American Vocational
  Association
  arteriovenous anastomosis

AV/AF
  anteverted, anteflexed

AVC
  allantoin vaginal cream
  associative visual cortex

AVC *(continued)*
    atrioventricular canal
    automatic volume control

AVCS
    atrioventricular
        conduction system

AVD
    aortic valve disease
    apparent volume of
        distribution
    arteriovenous difference

$AVDO_2$
    arteriovenous oxygen
        difference

avdp.
    avoirdupois

AVE
    aortic valve
        electrocardiogram

AVF
    antiviral factor
    arteriovenous fistula

aVF
    augmented unipolar lead,
        left leg

avg
    average

AVH
    acute viral hepatitis

AVI
    air velocity index

aVL
    augmented unipolar lead,
        left arm

AVM
    arteriovenous
        malformation
    atrioventricular
        malformation

AVMA
    American Veterinary
        Medical Association

AVN
    atrioventricular node
    avascular necrosis

AVP
    antiviral protein
    arginine vasopressin
    dactinomycin, vincristine,
        and cisplatin

AVR
    aortic valve replacement

aVR
    augmented unipolar lead,
        right arm

AVRP
    atrioventricular refractory
        period

AVS
    arteriovenous shunt

A-V shunt
    arteriovenous shunt

AVT
    Allen vision test
    area ventralis of Tsai
    arginine vasotocin

AW
    above waist
    anterior wall
    atomic warfare
    atomic weight

aw
    airways

A/W
    in accordance with

A&W
    alive and well

AWF
    adrenal weight factor

AWI
anterior wall infarction

AWMI
anterior wall myocardial infarction

AWOL
absent without leave

AWP
airway pressure

AWRS
anti-whole rabbit serum

awu
atomic weight unit

Ax
axillary

ax
axial
axillary

ax.
axillary
axis

axFem
axillofemoral bypass

ax grad
axial gradient

AXT
alternating exotropia

AYF
antiyeast factor

AYP
autolyzed yeast protein

Az
F. azote (nitrogen)

AZA
azathioprine

5-Aza
5-azacytidine

azg
azaguanine

AZQ
aziridinylbenzoquinone

AZS
automatic zero set

AZT
Aschheim-Zondek test
zidovudine
(azidothymidine)

AZ test
Aschheim-Zondek test

AzU
6-azauracil

5-AzU
5-azauracil

6-AzU
6-azauracil

AZUR
6-azauridine

AzUR
6-azauridine

5-AzUR
5-azauridine

6-AzUR
6-azauridine

B
bacillus
Baumé's scale
bel
Benoist's scale
bicuspid
(whole) blood
boron
buccal

B✓
billing info posted

B
Brucella
magnetic flux density

b
L. balneum (bath)
barn
base (in nucleic acid
sequencing)
born

β
β chain of hemoglobin

b.
L. bis (twice)

BA
Bachelor of Arts
backache
bacterial agglutination
betamethasone acetate
blocking antibody
bone age
bovine albumin
brachial artery
bronchial asthma
buccoaxial

B > A
bone greater than air

Ba
barium

Bab
Babinski

BAC
blood alcohol concentration
buccoaxiocervical

BACON
bleomycin, doxorubicin,
lomustine, vincristine,
and mechlorethamine

BACOP
bleomycin, doxorubicin,
cyclophosphamide,
vincristine, and
prednisone

Bact.
Bacterium

BaE
barium enema

BAEE
benzoyl arginine ethyl
ester
benzylarginine ethyl ester

BAEP
brainstem auditory evoked
potential

BAER
brainstem auditory evoked
response

BAG
buccoaxiogingival

BAIB
beta-aminoisobutyric acid

BAL
bronchoalveolar lavage
dimercaprol (British
antilewisite)

bal
balance
L. balneum (bath)

43

BALB
> binaural alternate loudness balance (test)

B-ALL
> B-cell acute lymphoblastic leukemia

BALT
> bronchus-associated lymphoid tissue

BaM
> barium meal

BAME
> benzoylarginine methyl ester

BAN
> British Approved Name

BAO
> basal acid output

BAP
> blood agar plate

BAPP
> bleomycin, doxorubicin, cisplatin, and prednisone

BAS
> British Anatomical Society

BASH
> body acceleration given synchronously with the heartbeat

basos
> basophils

BB
> bed bath
> blanket bath
> blood bank
> blood buffer base
> blue bloaters (emphysema)
> both bones
> breakthrough bleeding
> breast biopsy
> buffer base

BBA
> born before arrival

BBB
> blood-brain barrier
> bundle branch block

BBBB
> bilateral bundle branch block

BB to MM
> belly button to medial malleolus (examination)

BBOT
> 2,5-bis(5-*t*-butylbenzoxazol-2--yl) thiophene

BBSO
> black braided silk out (removed)

BBS(S)
> black braided silk (suture)

BBT
> basal body temperature

BC
> bactericidal concentration
> birth control
> bone conduction
> Bowman's capsule
> buccocervical

B&C
> bed and chair

BCAA
> branched-chain amino acid

BCAF
> basophil chemotaxis augmentation factor

B-CAVe
> bleomycin, lomustine, doxorubicin, and vinblastine

BCB
> brilliant cresyl blue

BC/BS
Blue Cross/Blue Shield

BCC
birth control clinic

BCD
binary coded decimal

BCDF
B cell differentiation
factors

BCE
basal cell epithelioma

B cell
bone marrow or bursa of
Fabricius derived cell

BCF
basophil chemotactic factor

BCG
bacille Calmette-Guérin
ballistocardiogram
bicolor guaiac test
bromcresol green

BCGF
B cell growth factors

B-CLL
B-cell chronic lymphatic
leukemia

BCLS
Basic Cardiac Life Support

BCM
birth control medication

BCNU
bischlorethylnitrosourea
bischloronitrosourea
carmustine

BCP
birth control pills
bromcresol purple

BCP-D
bromcresol purple
desoxycholate

BCRC
Baltimore Cancer Research
Center

BCTF
Breast Cancer Task Force

BCVPP
carmustine,
cyclophosphamide,
vinblastine, procarbazine,
and prednisone

BD
base deficit
base down
bile duct
buccodistal

b.d.
L. bis die (twice a day)

BDA
British Dental Association

BDC
burn-dressing change

BDG
buffered desoxycholate
glucose

B-DOPA
bleomycin, dacarbazine,
vincristine, prednisone,
and doxorubicin

BDS
Bachelor of Dental Surgery
British Dental Society

b.d.s.
L. bis die sumendum (to be
taken twice a day)

BDSc
Bachelor of Dental Science

BE
bacillary emulsion
(tuberculin)
bacterial endocarditis
barium enema

BE *(continued)*
  base excess
  bovine enteritis

B-E
  below the elbow
    (amputation)

Be
  beryllium

Bé
  Baumé

BEAM
  carmustine, etoposide,
    cytarabine, and
    melphalan

BEE
  basal energy expenditure

BEI
  butanol-extractable iodine

BEP
  bleomycin, etoposide,
    cisplatin

beta HCG
  pregnancy test using blood
    sample

BEV
  billion electron volts

BeV
  billion electron volts

Bev
  billion electron volts

bev
  billion electron volts

BF
  blastogenic factor
  blood flow
  breakfast fed

B/F
  bound-free ratio

bf
  bouillon filtrate
    (tuberculin)

BFC
  benign febrile convulsion

BFP
  biologic false-positive

BFR
  biologic false-positive
    reactor
  blood flow rate
  bone formation rate

BFT
  bentonite flocculation test

BFU-E
  burst forming
    units-erythroid

BG
  blood glucose
  bone graft
  buccogingival

B-G
  Bordet-Gengou (bacillus)

BGG
  bovine gamma globulin

BGH
  bovine growth hormone

BGP
  beta-glycerophosphatase

BGSA
  blood granulocyte-specific
    activity

BGTT
  borderline glucose
    tolerance test

BH
  benzalkonium and heparin
  bundle of His

BHA
  butylated hydroxyanisole

BHC
benzene hexachloride

BHCDA
Bureau of Health Care Delivery and Assistance

BHI
brain-heart infusion

BHK
baby hamster kidney

BHN
Brinell hardness number

BHPR
Bureau of Health Professions

BHRD
Bureau of Health Resources Development

BHS
beta-hemolytic streptococcus

BHT
butylated hydroxytoluene

BH/VH
body hematocrit-venous hematocrit ratio

BI
bacteriological index
base in
burn index

Bi
bismuth

Bib.
L. bibe (drink)

BID
brought in dead

b.i.d.
L. bis in die (twice a day)

BIDLB
block in the posteroinferior division of the left branch

BIDS
brittle hair, impaired intelligence, decreased fertility, and short stature

BIH
benign intracranial hypertension

BIL
bilateral

Bil
bilirubin

bilat
bilateral

BIN
L. bis in nocte (twice a night)

b.i.n.
L. bis in nocte (twice a night)

biol
biological

BIOS
British Intelligence Objectives Subcommittee

BIP
bismuth iodoform paste

BiP]
immunoglobulin-binding protein

BIS
twice

BJ
Bence Jones
biceps jerk

B&J
bone and joint

BJM
bones, joints, and muscles

BJP
> Bence Jones protein

BK
> below the knee

B-K
> below the knee
> (amputation)

Bk
> berkelium

BKA
> below knee amputation

bkft
> breakfast

bkfst
> breakfast

BKV
> BK virus

BKWP
> below knee walking plaster

BL
> baseline
> Bessey-Lowry (units)
> bleeding
> blood loss
> buccolingual
> Burkitt's lymphoma

BLB
> Boothby, Lovelace,
> Bulbulian (mask)

BLB mask
> Boothby-Lovelace-Bulbulian
> mask

BLB unit
> Bessey-Lowry-Brock unit

bl cult
> blood culture

BLE
> bilateral lower extremity

BLEO
> bleomycin sulfate

Bleo
> bleomycin sulfate

BLG
> beta-lactoglobulin

BLN
> bronchial lymph nodes

bl pr
> blood pressure

BLS
> basic life support

BLT
> blood-clot lysis time

BLU
> Bessey-Lowry units

BLV
> bovine leukemia virus

BM
> L. balneum maris
> (seawater bath)
> basement membrane
> body mass
> bone marrow
> bone mass
> bowel movement
> buccomesial

BMA
> British Medical
> Association

BME
> brief maximal effort

BMG
> benign monoclonal
> gammopathy
> beta$_2$-microglobulin

BMI
> body mass index

BMJ
> British Medical Journal

bmk
> birthmark

B-mod
> behavior modification

B-mode
> brightness modulation

BMP
> bleomycin, methotrexate, and cisplatin
> bone marrow pressure

BMR
> basal metabolic rate

BMS
> Bachelor of Medical Science

BMT
> bone marrow transplantation

BMU
> basic multicellular unit

BN
> brachial neuritis

BNA
> Basle Nomina Anatomica

BNC
> bladder neck contracture

BNO
> bladder neck obstruction

BNPA
> binasal pharyngeal airway

BNS
> benign nephrosclerosis

BO
> base of prism out
> body odor
> bowel obstruction
> bucco-occlusal

B&O
> belladonna and opium

BOA
> born on arrival
> British Orthopaedic Association

BOBA
> beta-oxybutyric acids

BOC
> former abbreviation for *t*-butoxycarbonyl (current usage is Boc)

***t*-BOC**
> former abbreviation for *t*-butoxycarbonyl (current usage is Boc)

Boc
> *t*-butoxycarbonyl

BOD
> biochemical oxygen demand

Bod Units
> Bodansky units

BOEA
> ethyl biscoumacetate

BOH
> bundle of His

boil
> boiling

Bol.
> L. bolus (pill)

BOLD
> bleomycin, vincristine, lomustine, and dacarbazine

BOM
> bilateral otitis media

BOOP
> bronchiolitis obliterans with organizing pneumonia

BOPP
bleomycin sulfate, vincristine, procarbazine, and prednisone

BOW
bag of waters

BP
back pressure
bathroom privileges
bedpan
benzopyrene
birthplace
blood pressure
British Pharmacopoeia
bronchopleural
buccopulpal
bypass

bp
base pair

b.p.
boiling point

BPA
in Tanner staging: breast, pubic, axillary hair
British Paediatric Association

BPC
British Pharmaceutical Codex

BPD
biparietal diameter
bronchopulmonary dysplasia

BPEAOA
Bureau of Professional Education of the American Osteopathic Association

BPH
benign prostatic hypertrophy

B Ph
British Pharmacopoeia

BPIG
bacterial polysaccharide immune globulin

BPL
beta-propiolactone

BPM
beats per minute

BPO
benzylpenicilloyl

BPRS
brief psychiatric rating scale

BPS
Baseline Prevalence Survey

BPV
bovine papilloma virus

Bq
becquerel

BR
bathroom
bedrest
bilirubin
British or Birmingham Revision (of BNA terminology)

Br
bromine

Br
Brucella

br
bromo

BRAT
bananas, rice cereal, applesauce, and toast

BRBC
bovine red blood cells

BrdU
bromodeoxyuridine

BRFSS

    Behavioral Risk Factor
    Surveillance System

Brit

    Britain
    British

BRM

    biological response
      modifier
    biuret-reactive material

BRP

    bathroom privileges
    bilirubin production
    British Roentgen Society

b.r.p.

    bathroom privileges

brth

    breath

BS

    Bachelor of Science
    Bachelor of Surgery
    blood sugar
    Blue Shield
    bowel sounds
    breath sounds

B&S

    Bartholin and Skene's
      (glands)

BSA

    bismuth-sulfite agar
    body surface area
    bovine serum albumin

BSAP

    brief short-action potential

BSB

    body surface burned

BSDLB

    block in the anterosuperior
      division of the left branch

BSE

    bilateral symmetrical and
      equal

BSE *(continued)*

    breast self-examination

BSER

    brain stem-evoked
      response

BSF

    backscatter factor

BSF-2

    B cell stimulatory factor 2

BSI

    bound serum iron

BSL

    blood sugar level

BSN

    Bachelor of Science in
      Nursing
    bowel sounds normal

BSO

    bilateral
      salpingo-oophorectomy
    buthionine sulfoximine

BSP

    Bromsulphalein

BSR

    basal skin resistance

BSS

    balanced salt solution
    black silk suture
    buffered saline solution

BST

    brief stimulus therapy

BSU

    British standard units

BT

    bedtime
    bladder tumor
    bleeding time
    brain tumor

BTB

    breakthrough bleeding

BTE
Baltimore Therapeutic Equipment Work Simulator

BThU
British thermal unit

BTL
bilateral tubal ligation

BTLS
basic trauma life support

BTPS
gas volume expressed as if it were saturated with water vapor at body temperature and at the ambient barometric pressure

BTSG
Brain Tumor Study Group

BTU
British thermal unit

BU
base of prism up
Bodansky unit
burn unit

Bu
butyl

BUDR
5-bromodeoxyuridine

BUE
bilateral upper extremity

Bull.
L. bulliat (let it boil)

BUN
blood urea nitrogen

BUPA
British United Provident Association

BUS
Bartholin's, urethral, and Skene's glands

But.
L. butyrum (butter)

BV
biological value
blood vessel
blood volume
bronchovesicular
vapor bath (balneum vaporis)

BVH
biventricular hypertrophy

BVI
blood vessel invasion

BVR
Bureau of Vocational Rehabilitation

BVV
bovine vaginitis virus

BW
birth weight
body water
body weight

Bx
biopsy

bx
biopsy

BYE
Barile-Yaguchi-Eveland (culture medium)

Bz
benzoyl

bz
benzoyl

Bza
benzimidazole
benzimidazolyl

BzAnth
benzanthracene

BzH
benzaldehyde

bzl
   benzyl

BzOH
   benzoic acid

C
calculus
calorie
carbohydrate
carbon
cathodal
cathode
Caucasian
Celsius
centigrade
L. centum (hundred)
cervical vertebrae (C1–C7)
chest
clearance
clonus
closure
color sense
communicating
  (pacemaker code)
complement (C1–C9)
compound
contraction
contracture
coulomb
curie
cylinder
cytidine
cytosine
hematocrit
hundred
speed of light

C.
L. congius (gallon)

C
capacitance
clearance
Clostridium
Cryptococcus

°C
degree Celsius

C_{II}
second cranial nerve

C_{alb}
albumin clearance

C_{am}
amylase clearance

C_{cr}
creatinine clearance

C_H
constant region of an
  immunoglobulin heavy
  chain

C_{in}
insulin clearance

C_L
constant region of an
  immunoglobulin light
  chain

C_p
heat capacity

C_{pah}
para-aminohippurate
  clearance

C_u
urea clearance

C′
symbol for complement

ⓒ
confidential (patient may
  be unaware)

C§
cesarean section

c
capillary
centi-
contact
curie
small calorie

c.
L. cibus (food)
L. cum (with)

55

c
> molar concentration
> specific heat capacity
> velocity of light in a
> vacuum

$\bar{c}$
> L. cum (with)

c'
> coefficient of partage

CA
> cancer
> carbonic anhydrase
> carcinoma
> cardiac arrest
> cathode
> cervicoaxial
> Chemical Abstracts
> chronologic age
> cold agglutinins
> common antigen
> coronary artery
> corpora amylacea
> croup-associated (virus)
> cyclophosphamide,
> doxorubicin

(CA)n
> contain

Ca
> calcium
> cancer
> Cancer - A Cancer Journal
> for Clinicians
> carcinoma
> carpal
> carpal amputation
> cathodal
> cathode
> NIOSH recommends that
> the substance be treated
> as a potential human
> carcinogen

ca
> cancer

ca.
> L. circa (about)

CAA
> carotid audiofrequency
> analysis

CAAT
> computer-assisted axial
> tomography

CAB
> coronary artery bypass

CABG
> coronary artery bypass
> graft

CACC
> cathodal closure
> contraction

CaCC
> cathodal closure
> contraction

CACMS
> Committee on
> Accreditation of
> Canadian Medical
> Schools

$CaCO_3$
> calcium carbonate

CAD
> coronary artery disease

CaDTe
> cathodal duration tetanus

CAE
> cellulose acetate
> electrophoresis

CaEDTA
> calcium disodium edetate

CAF
> cyclophosphamide,
> doxorubicin, and
> 5-fluorouracil

CAFT
cisplatin, doxorubicin, 5-fluorouracil, and teniposide

CAG
chronic atrophic gastritis

CAH
chronic active hepatitis
chronic aggressive hepatitis
congenital adrenal hyperplasia

CAHD
coronary atherosclerotic heart disease

CAHEA (AMA)
Committee on Allied Health Education and Accreditation

Cal
large calorie (kilocalorie)

cal
calorie

calc
calculate

calcd
calculated

Calef.
L. calefac (make warm)
L. calefactus (warmed)

CALGB
cancer and leukemia group B

CALLA
common acute lymphoblastic leukemia antigen

CAM
chorioallantoic membrane
contralateral axillary metastasis

CAMP
cyclophosphamide, doxorubicin, methotrexate, and procarbazine

cAMP
cyclic adenosine monophosphate

CANCERLIT
an electronic database including citations relating to oncology

CAO
chronic airway obstruction

CaOC
cathodal opening contraction

CaOCl
cathodal opening clonus

CAP
capsule
catabolite activator protein
cellulose acetate phthalate
chloramphenicol
cyclophosphamide, doxorubicin, and cisplatin
cystine aminopeptidase

Cap.
L. capiat (let him take)

cap
capsule

cap.
L. capsula (capsule)

CAPD
continuous ambulatory peritoneal dialysis

Capsul.
L. capsula (capsule)

CAR
Canadian Association of Radiologists

CARF
    Commission on Accreditation of Rehabilitation Facilities

CAS
    Chemical Abstracts Service
    Council of Academic Societies

CASS
    Coronary Artery Surgery Study

CAT
    Children's Apperception Test
    chloramphenicol acetyltransferase
    chlormerodrin accumulation test
    computed axial tomography
    computerized axial tomography

CAT-CAM
    contoured adducted trochanteric-controlled alignment method

Cath.
    L. catharticus (cathartic)

cath
    catheter
    catheterization

CATS
    combined abdominal transsacral resection technique

CAV
    congenital absence of vagina
    congenital adrenal virilism
    cyclophosphamide, doxorubicin, and vincristine

CAVB
    complete atrioventricular block

CAVmP
    cyclophosphamide, doxorubicin, teniposide, and prednisone

CAVP
    lomustine, melphalan, etoposide, and prednisone

CAWO
    closing abductory wedge osteotomy

CB
    L. Chirurgiae Baccalaureus (Bachelor of Surgery)
    chronic bronchitis
    contrast baths

Cb
    symbol for columbium

CBA
    chronic bronchitis with asthma

CBB
    Coomassie brilliant blue

CBC
    complete blood count

cbc
    complete blood count

CBD
    closed bladder drainage
    common bile duct

CBF
    cerebral blood flow
    coronary blood flow

CBG
    corticosteroid-binding globulin
    cortisol-binding globulin

CBI
  continuous bladder
    irrigation

Cbl
  cobalamin

CBPP
  contagious bovine
    pleuropneumonia

CBR
  complete bed rest

CBS
  chronic brain syndrome

CBV
  central blood volume
  circulating blood volume
  corrected blood volume
  cyclophosphamide,
    carmustine, and etoposide

Cbz
  carbobenzoxy
    (benzyloxycarbonyl)

CC
  cardiac cycle
  chief complaint
  circulatory collapse
  colony count
  compound cathartic
  coracoclavicular
  cord compression
  corpus callosum
  costochondral
  creatinine clearance
  critical condition

cc
  cubic centimeter

c̄c
  with meals

CCA
  chick-cell agglutination
  chimpanzee coryza agent
    (respiratory syncytial
    virus)

CCA *(continued)*
  common carotid artery
  congenital contractural
    arachnodactyly

CCAT
  conglutinating complement
    absorption test

CCC
  cathodal closure
    contraction
  chronic calculous
    cholecystitis

CCCl
  cathodal closure clonus

CCDPHP
  Center for Chronic Disease
    Prevention and Health
    Promotion

CCE
  clubbing, cyanosis, and
    edema

CCF
  cephalin-cholesterol
    flocculation
  compound comminuted
    fracture
  congestive cardiac failure
  crystal-induced
    chemotactic factor

CCI
  chronic coronary
    insufficiency

CCK
  cholecystokinin

CCK-PZ
  cholecystokinin-pancreozy-
    min

CCM
  critical care medicine

c cm
  cubic centimeter

CCME
Coordinating Council on
Medical Education

CCMSU
clean catch midstream
urine

CCNU
lomustine

Ccnu
lomustine

CCP
ciliocytophthoria

Ccr
creatinine clearance

CCRN
Critical Care Registered
Nurse

CCS
Cronkhite-Canada
syndrome

CCSG
Children's Cancer Study
Group

CCTe
cathodal closure tetanus

CCU
Cherry-Crandall units
coronary care unit

CCV
conductivity cell volume

CCW
counterclockwise

CD
cadaver donor
cardiac disease
cardiac dullness
cardiovascular disease
caudal
cesarean delivered
circular dichroism
cluster designation

CD *(continued)*
common duct
compact optical disk
L. conjugata diagonalis
(diagonal conjugate
diameter)
consanguineous donor
convulsive disorder
curative dose
cystic duct

Cd
cadmium
coccygeal

cd
candela

C&D
cystoscopy and dilatation

C/D
cigarettes per day

CDA
chenodeoxycholic acid
congenital
dyserythropoietic anemia

CDB
cough and deep breath

C&DB
cough and deep breath

CDC
calculated date of
confinement
Centers for Disease Control
chenodeoxycholic acid

CDC/AIDS
Centers for Disease Control
definition of acquired
immunodeficiency
syndrome

CDD
certificate of disability for
discharge

CDE
blood group antigen (Rh
system)

CDE *(continued)*
    canine distemper
      encephalitis
    chlordiazepoxide
    common duct exploration

cdf
    cumulative distribution
      function

CDGP
    constitutional delay of
      growth and puberty

CDH
    ceramide dihexoside
    congenital dislocation of
      hip
    congenitally dysplastic hip

CDI
    Cotrel-Dubousset
      instrumentation

CDL
    chlorodeoxylincomycin

cDNA
    complementary DNA
    copy DNA

CDP
    continuous distending
      pressure
    cytidine diphosphate

CDS
    cul-de-sac

cdyn
    dynamic compliance

CE
    California encephalitis
    cardiac enlargement
    chick embryo
    cholesterol esters
    contractile element

Ce
    cerium

CEA
    carcinoembryonic antigen

CEA *(continued)*
    crystalline egg albumin

CEEV
    Central European
      encephalitis virus

CEF
    chick embryo fibroblast

Cel
    Celsius

p-CMB

Cels
    Celsius

CEM
    lomustine, etoposide, and
      methotrexate

CEN
    Certified Emergency Nurse

CEP
    congenital erythropoietic
      porphyria
    countercurrent
      electrophoresis
    lomustine, etoposide, and
      prednimustine

CER
    ceruloplasmin
    conditioned emotional
      response
    conditioned escape
      response

Cer
    ceramide

cerv
    cervical

ces
    central excitatory state

CESD
    cholesteryl ester storage
      disease

CEU
    continuing education unit

CEVD

lomustine, etoposide, vindesine, and dexamethasone

CF

antibody titer
calibration factor
cancer-free
carbolfuchsin
cardiac failure
carrier-free
chemotactic factor
chest and left leg
Chiari-Frommel syndrome
Christmas factor
citrovorum factor
complement fixation
contractile force
count fingers
cystic fibrosis

Cf

californium

cf

L. confer (bring together, compare)

CFA

complement-fixating antibody
complete Freund's adjuvant

CFF

critical flicker fusion test

cff

critical fusion frequency

CFMG

Commission on Foreign Medical Graduates

CFP

chronic false-positive
cyclophosphamide, 5-fluorouracil, and prednisone
cystic fibrosis of the pancreas

CFPMV

cyclophosphamide, 5-fluorouracil, prednisone, methotrexate, and vincristine

CFPT

cyclophosphamide, 5-fluorouracil, prednisone, and tamoxifen

CFR

Code of Federal Regulations

CFT

complement-fixation test

CFU

colony-forming unit

CFU-C

colony-forming unit–culture

CFU-E

colony-forming unit–erythroid

CFU/mL

colony-forming units/mL

CFU-S

colony-forming unit–spleen

CFWM

cancer-free white mouse

CG

Cardio-Green
chorionic gonadotropin
chronic glomerulonephritis
colloidal gold
phosgene (choking gas)

cg

centigram

CGA

catabolite gene activator
chromogranin-A

CGD
 chronic granulomatous
 disease

CGFNS
 Commission on Graduates
 of Foreign Nursing
 Schools

cgi
 clinical global impression

CGL
 chronic granulocytic
 leukemia
 correction with glasses

cgm
 centigram

cGMP
 cyclic guanosine
 monophosphate

CGN
 chronic glomerulonephritis

CGNA
 Canadian Gerontological
 Nursing Association

CG/OQ
 cerebral glucose oxygen
 quotient

CGP
 choline glycerophosphatide
 chorionic growth hormone
 prolactin
 circulating granulocyte
 pool

CGPM
 Conférence Générale des
 Poids et Mesures

CGS
 centimeter-gram-second

cgs
 centimeter-gram-second

CGT
 chorionic gonadotropin

CGTT
 cortisone glucose tolerance
 test

cGy
 centigray

CH
 cholesterol
 crown-heel (length of fetus)

CH_{50}
 total serum hemolytic
 complement

Ch
 chapter

Ch^1
 Christchurch chromosome

ch
 chest

ch^1
 Christchurch chromosome

CH50
 total serum hemolytic
 complement

CHA
 congenital hypoplastic
 anemia
 cyclohexylamine

CHAC
 cyclophosphamide,
 hexamethylmelamine,
 doxorubicin, and
 carboplatin

CHAD
 cyclophosphamide,
 hexamethylmelamine,
 doxorubicin, and cisplatin

CHAMOCA
 cyclophosphamide,
 hydroxyurea,
 dactinomycin,
 methotrexate, vincristine,
 and doxorubicin

CHAMPUS
    Civilian Health and
        Medical Program of the
        Uniformed Services

CHAP
    cyclophosphamide,
        hexamethylmelamine,
        doxorubicin, and cisplatin

chart.
    L. charta (paper)

CHB
    complete heart block

Ch.B.
    L. Chirurgiae Baccalaureus
        (Bachelor of Surgery)

CHD
    childhood disease
    congenital heart disease
    congestive heart disease
    coronary heart disease

ChD
    L. Chirurgiae Doctor
        (Doctor of Surgery)

ChE
    cholinesterase

Chem
    chemotherapy

chem
    chemical
    chemistry

ChemoRx
    chemotherapy

CHF
    congestive heart failure
    cyclophosphamide,
        hexamethylmelamine,
        and 5-fluorouracil

CHH
    cartilage-hair hypoplasia

CHINA
    chronic infectious
        neuropathic (or
        neurotropic) agent

CHL
    chlorambucil
    chloramphenicol

Chl
    chlorambucil

ChlVPP
    chlorambucil, vinblastine,
        procarbazine, and
        prednisone

ChM
    L. Chirurgiae Magister
        (Master of Surgery)

CHMD
    clinical hyaline membrane
        disease

CHN
    central hemorrhagic
        necrosis

CHO
    carbohydrate
    Chinese hamster ovary
    cyclophosphamide,
        doxorubicin, and
        vincristine

Cho
    choline

Chol
    cholesterol

chol
    cholesterol

CHOP
    cyclophosphamide,
        doxorubicin, vincristine,
        and prednisone

CHOP-B
cyclophosphamide, doxorubicin, vincristine, prednisone, and bleomycin

CHOP-BLEO
bleomycin, cyclophosphamide, doxorubicin, vincristine, and prednisone

CHPX
chickenpox

chpx
chickenpox

chr
chronic

Chr.
Chromobacterium

CHS
Chédiak-Higashi syndrome
cholinesterase
contact hypersensitivity

CI
cardiac index
cardiac insufficiency
cerebral infarction
chemotherapeutic index
colloidal iron
color index
Colour Index
confidence interval
continuous infusion
coronary insufficiency
crystalline insulin

Ci
curie

CIB
Current Intelligence Bulletin

Cib.
L. cibus (food)

CICU
coronary (cardiac) intensive care unit

CID
cytomegalic inclusion disease

CIDS
cellular immunodeficiency syndrome

CIE
counterimmunoelectrophoresis
countercurrent immunoelectrophoresis

CIEP
counterimmunoelectrophoresis

CIF
clonal inhibitory factor

cig
cigarettes

CIH
Certificate in Industrial Health

Ci-hr
curie-hour

CIN
cefsulodin-irgasan-novobiocin (agar)
cervical intraepithelial neoplasia
chronic interstitial nephritis

circ
circulation
circumcision

CIS
carcinoma in situ
central inhibitory state

cis-DDP
cisplatin

CIXU
constant infusion excretory urogram

CJD
Creutzfeldt-Jakob disease

CK
check
creatine kinase

CKD
Creutzfeldt-Jakob disease

C/kg
coulomb per kilogram

CL
chest and left arm
critical list

Cl
chloride
chlorine

Cl
Clostridium

cl
centiliter
corpus luteum

CLAS
congenital localized absence of skin

CLBBB
complete left bundle branch block

CL/CP
cleft lip and cleft palate

CLD
chronic liver disease
chronic lung disease

CLH
chronic lobular hepatitis

ClHgBzO
chloromercuribenzoate

clin
clinic

clin *(continued)*
clinical

CLIP
corticotropin-like intermediate lobe peptide

CLL
chronic lymphatic leukemia
chronic lymphocytic leukemia

CLMA
Clinical Laboratory Management Association

CLO
cod liver oil

CLQ
cognitive laterality quotient

CLSH
corpus luteum-stimulating hormone

CLSL
chronic lymphosarcoma (cell) leukemia

CLT
clot-lysis time

ClT
total plasma clearance

CM
capreomycin
cardiac monitor
L. Chirurgiae Magister (Master of Surgery)
chloroquine-mepacrine
cochlear microphonics
costal margin
cow's milk

C.M.
L. cras mane (tomorrow morning)

Cm
curium

cM
  centimorgan

cm
  centimeter

cm^2
  square centimeter

cm^3
  cubic centimeter

CMA
  California Medical
    Association
  Canadian Medical
    Association
  Certified Medical Assistant
  Chinese Medical
    Association

CMAJ
  Canadian Medical
    Association Journal

CMAP
  compound muscle action
    potential

CMB
  carbolic methylene blue

p-CMB
  para-chloromercuribenzoate-

CMC
  carboxymethylcellulose
  carpometacarpal
  critical micelle
    concentration

CM-cellulose
  carboxymethylcellulose

CMD
  cerebromacular
    degeneration
  Current Medical Dialog

CME
  continuing medical
    education
  Council on Medical
    Education

CMF
  chondromyxoid fibroma
  cyclophosphamide
    (Cytoxan), methotrexate,
    and 5-fluorouracil

CMFP
  cyclophosphamide,
    methotrexate,
    5-fluorouracil, and
    prednisone

CMFVP
  cyclophosphamide,
    methotrexate,
    5-fluorouracil,
    vincristine, and
    prednisone

CMG
  cystometrogram

CMGN
  chronic membranous
    glomerulonephritis

CMHC
  community mental health
    center

CMI
  carbohydrate metabolism
    index
  cell-mediated immunity

CMID
  cytomegalic inclusion
    disease

c/min
  cycles per minute

CML
  cell-mediated
    lymphocytotoxicity
  cell-mediated lympholysis
  chronic myelocytic
    leukemia
  chronic myelogenous
    leukemia

CMM
cutaneous malignant melanoma

c mm
cubic millimeter

CMN
cystic medial necrosis

CMN-AA
cystic medial necrosis of the ascending aorta

CMO
calculated mean organism
cardiac minute output

cMo
centimorgan

CMoL
chronic monocytic (monoblastic) leukemia

C-MOPP
cyclophosphamide, mechlorethamine, vincristine, procarbazine, and prednisone

CMOS
complementary metal oxide semiconductor

CMP
cardiomyopathy
cytidine monophosphate

CMR
cerebral metabolic rate
crude mortality rate

CMRG
cerebral metabolic rate of glucose

CMRNG
chromosomally resistant *Neisseria gonorrhoeae*

CMRO
cerebral metabolic rate of oxygen

CMRO$_2$
cerebral metabolic rate of oxygen

CMRR
common mode rejection ratio

CMS
circulation, muscle sensation
Clyde Mood Scale

c.m.s.
L. cras mane sumendus (to be taken tomorrow morning)

CMSS
Council of Medical Specialty Societies

CMT
Certified Medical Transcriptionist
circus movement tachycardia

CMU
chlorophenyldimethylurea

CMV
cisplatin, methotrexate, and vinblastine
cytomegalovirus

CN
cranial nerve
cyanide anion
cyanogen
L. cras nocte (tomorrow night)

CNA
Canadian Nurses Association

CN-Cbl
cyanocobalamin

CNE
chronic nervous exhaustion

CNHD
congenital nonspherocytic hemolytic disease

CNL
cardiolipin natural lecithin

CNM
Certified Nurse-Midwife

CNP
continuous negative pressure

CNRRA
Chinese National Relief and Rehabilitation Administration

CNS
central nervous system

c.n.s.
L. cras nocte sumendus (to be taken tomorrow night)

CNV
conative negative variation
contingent negative variation

CO
carbon monoxide
cardiac output
castor oil
centric occlusion
cervicoaxial
coenzyme
compound
corneal opacity

C/O
check out
complains of

CO_2
carbon dioxide

Co
cobalt

COA
Canadian Orthopaedic Association

CoA
coenzyme A

COAD
chronic obstructive airway disease

coag
coagulation

COAP
cyclophosphamide, vincristine, cytarabine, prednisone

CoA-SH
coenzyme A

COBMAM
cyclophosphamide, vincristine, bleomycin, methotrexate, doxorubicin, and semustine

COBS
cesarean-obtained barrier-sustained

COBT
chronic obstruction of biliary tract

COC
calcifying odontogenic cyst
cathodal opening clonus
cathodal opening contraction
coccygeal

cochl.
L. cochleare (a spoonful)

cochl. amp.
L. cochleare amplum (a heaping spoonful)

cochl. mag.
L. cochleare magnum (a tablespoonful)

cochl. med.
  L. cochleare medium (a
    dessertspoonful)

cochl. parv.
  L. cochleare parvum (a
    teaspoonful)

COCl
  cathodal opening clonus

coct.

Coct.
  L. coctio (boiling)

COD
  cause of death

cod.
  codeine

COEAMRA
  Council on Education of
    the American Medical
    Record Association

coef
  coefficient

coeff
  coefficient

COG
  Central Oncology Group

COGTT
  cortisone-primed oral
    glucose tolerance test

COH
  carbohydrate

COHb
  carboxyhemoglobin

Col.
  L. cola (strain)

Colat.
  L. colatus (strained)

COLD
  chronic obstructive lung
    disease

Colet.
  L. coletur (let it be
    strained)

coll.
  L. collyrium (eyewash)

coll
  college

collat
  collateral

Collut.
  L. collutorium
    (mouth-wash)

coll. vol.
  collective volume

Collyr.
  L. collyrium (eyewash)

Color.
  L. coloretur (let it be
    colored)

COMLA
  cyclophosphamide,
    vincristine, methotrexate,
    leucovorin, and
    cytarabine

comm.
  committee

commn.
  commission
  commissioner

COMP
  cyclophosphamide,
    vincristine, methotrexate,
    and prednisone

Comp.
  L. compositus (compound)

compd
  compound

complic
  complicating
  complication(s)

compn
  composition

COMT
  catechol-*o*-methyl-
    transferase

CON
  certificate of need

ConA
  concanavalin A

conc
  concentrated

Concis.
  L. concisus (cut)

concn
  concentration

conf
  conference

config
  configuration

cong.
  L. congius (gallon)

cong
  congress

congen
  congenital

Cons.
  L. conserva (keep)

const
  constant

constit
  constituent

Cont.
  L. contusus (bruised)

contd
  continued

contg
  containing

Contin.
  L. continuetur (let it be
    continued)

Cont. rem.
  L. continuetur remedium
    (let the medicine be
    continued)

COP
  colloid osmotic pressure
  cyclophosphamide,
    vincristine, and
    prednisone

COP-BLAM
  cyclophosphamide,
    vincristine, prednisone,
    bleomycin, doxorubicin,
    and procarbazine

COPD
  chronic obstructive
    pulmonary disease

COPE
  chronic obstructive
    pulmonary emphysema

COPP
  cyclophosphamide,
    vincristine, prednisone,
    and procarbazine

CoQ
  coenzyme Q

Coq.
  L. coque (boil)

Coq. in s. a.
  L. coque in sufficiente aqua
    (boil in sufficient water)

Coq. s. a.
  L. coque secundum artem
    (boil properly)

COR
  comprehensive outpatient
    rehabilitation facility
  heart

CORA
 conditioned orientation
  reflex audiometry

cor
 corrected

corr
 corrected

corresp
 corresponding

Cort.
 L. cortex (bark)

COS
 Canadian
  Ophthalmological Society

COTA
 Certified Occupational
  Therapy Assistant

COTe
 cathodal opening tetanus

COTH
 Council of Teaching
  Hospitals

CP
 candle power
 carotid pressure
 cerebral palsy
 chemically pure
 chest pain
 chloropurine
 chloroquine and
  primaquine (combination
  tablets)
 chronic pyelonephritis
 cleft palate
 closing pressure
 cochlear potential
 coproporphyrin
 creatine phosphokinase

C&P
 cystoscopy and
  pyelography

C/P
 cholesterol-phospholipid
  ratio

cp
 centipoise

CPA
 cerebellar pontine angle
 chlorophenylalanine
 cyclophosphamide

C3PA
 C3 proactivator

C3PAase
 C3 proactivator convertase

CPAN
 Certified Post Anesthesia
  Nurse

CPAP
 continuous positive airway
  pressure

CPB
 cardiopulmonary bypass
 competitive protein
  binding

CPC
 cetylpyridinium chloride
 chronic passive congestion
 clinicopathological
  conference
 cresolphthalein
  complexone

CPD
 cephalopelvic disproportion
 citrate phosphate dextrose
  compound

CPDA-1
 citrate phosphate dextrose
  adenine

CPDD
 calcium pyrophosphate
  deposition disease

CPE
  chronic pulmonary
    emphysema
  cytopathic effect

C Ped
  Certified Pedorthist

CPH
  Certificate in Public
    Health
  chronic persistent hepatitis

CPHA
  Committee on Professional
    and Hospital Activities

CP\I
  chest pain or indigestion

CPI
  coronary prognostic index

CPIB
  chlorophenoxyisobutyrate

CPK
  creatine phosphokinase

CPM
  continuous passive motion

cpm
  counts per minute

CPN
  chronic pyelonephritis

CPNA
  Certified Pediatric Nurses
    Association

CPNP
  Certified Pediatric Nurse
    Practitioner

CPP
  cerebral perfusion pressure
  cyclopentenophenanthrene

CPPB
  continuous positive
    pressure breathing

CPPD
  calcium pyrophosphate
    dihydrate
  calcium pyrophosphate
    dihydrate disease

CPPV
  continuous positive
    pressure ventilation

CPR
  cardiopulmonary
    resuscitation
  cerebral cortex perfusion
    rate
  cortisol production rate

CPS
  carbamoyl phosphate
    synthetase
  Center for Preventive
    Services
  Compendium of
    Pharmaceuticals and
    Specialties

CPSI
  carbamoyl phosphate
    synthetase I

CPS-I
  Cancer Prevention Study I

CPSII
  carbamoyl phosphate
    synthetase II

CPS-II
  Cancer Prevention Study II

cps
  cycles per second

CPT
  chest physiotherapy

CPU
  central processing unit (in
    a computer)

CPZ
  chlorpromazine

CQ
   chloroquine-quinine
   circadian quotient

CR
   cardiorespiratory
   chest and right arm
   chloride
   closed reduction
   cold recombinant
   colon resection
   complement receptor
   complete remission
   complete response
   conditioned reflex
   conditioned response
   creatinine
   crown-rump

CR_1
   first cranial nerve

Cr
   creatinine
   chromium

CRA
   central retinal artery

cran
   cranial

Crast.
   L. crastinus (for tomorrow)

CRBBB
   complete right bundle
      branch block

CRC
   colorectal cancer

CRCS
   Canadian Red Cross
      Society

CRD
   chronic renal disease
   chronic respiratory disease
   complete reaction of
      degeneration

CREAT
   creatinine

CREG
   cross-reactive group (of
      HLA antigens)

C region
   constant region

CREST
   calcinosis, Raynaud's
      phenomenon, esophageal
      motility disorders,
      sclerodactyly, and
      telangiectasia

CRF
   chronic renal failure
   corticotropin releasing
      factor

CRH
   corticotropin-releasing
      hormone

CRIE
   crossed
      immunoelectrophoresis

crit
   hematocrit

CRITOE
   capitellum, radial head,
      internal condyle,
      trochlea, olecranon,
      external condyle
      (ossification sequence in
      elbow)

crit press
   critical pressure

crit temp
   critical temperature

CRL
   crown-rump length

CRM
   Certified Reference
      Materials
   cross-reacting material

Crn
     corrin

CRNA
     Certified Registered Nurse
        Anesthetist

cr ns
     cranial nerves

CRO
     cathode ray oscilloscope

CROS
     contralateral routing of
        signals

CRP
     C-reactive protein

CRS
     Chinese restaurant
        syndrome
     colon-rectal surgery

CRST
     calcinosis cutis, Raynaud's
        phenomenon,
        sclerodactyly, and
        telangiectasia

CRT
     cathode ray tube

CRU
     clinical research unit

CRV
     central retinal vein

Crys.
     crystal

cryst
     crystalline
     crystallization

CS
     cesarean section
     chondroitin sulfate
     chorionic
        somatomammotropin
     clinical specialist
     clinical stage

CS *(continued)*
     clinical state
     colorimetric solution
     conditioned stimulus
     coronary sinus
     corpus striatum
     corticosteroid
     cycloserine

C&S
     conjunctiva and sclera
     culture & sensitivity

Cs
     cesium

c/s
     cycle(s) per second

CSA
     canavaninosuccinic acid
     chondroitin sulfate A
     colony-stimulating activity
     compressed spectral assay

CsA
     cyclosporin A

CSAA
     Child Study Association of
        America

CSC
     Fr. coup sur coup (in small
        doses at short intervals)

CSE
     control standard exotoxin

CSF
     cerebrospinal fluid
     colony-stimulating factor

CSF-1
     macrophage
        colony-stimulating factor

CSGBI
     Cardiac Society of Great
        Britain and Ireland

CSH
     chronic subdural
        hematoma

CSH *(continued)*
    cortical stromal
        hyperplasia

CSL
    cardiolipin synthetic
        lecithin

CSM
    cerebrospinal meningitis

CSN
    carotid sinus nerve

CSOM
    chronic suppurative otitis
        media

C-spine
    cervical spine

CSR
    Cheyne-Stokes respiration
    corrected sedimentation
        rate
    cortisol secretion rate

CSS
    carotid sinus stimulation
    chewing, sucking, and
        swallowing

CST
    contraction stress test
    convulsive shock therapy
    static compliance

cSt
    centistoke

CSU
    catheter specimen of urine

CT
    calcitonin
    cardiothoracic
    carotid tracing
    carpal tunnel
    cerebral thrombosis
    chemotherapy
    chlorothiazide
    circulation time
    clotting time
    coagulation time

CT *(continued)*
    collecting tubule
    computed tomography
    computerized tomography
    connective tissue
    contraction time
    Coombs' test
    corneal transplant
    coronary thrombosis
    corrected transposition
    corrective therapy
    counseling and testing
    crest time
    cytotechnologist

CTA
    Canadian Tuberculosis
        Association
    chromotropic acid

CTAB
    cetyltrimethylammonium
        bromide

CTAT
    computerized transaxial
        tomography

CTBA
    cetrimonium bromide

CTC
    chlortetracycline

CTD
    carpal tunnel
        decompression
    congenital thymic
        dysplasia

CTFA
    The Cosmetic, Toiletry,
        and Fragrance
        Association

CTFE
    chlorotrifluoroethylene

CTH
    ceramide trihexoside

CTL
    cytotoxic T lymphocytes

CTLp
cytotoxic T lymphocyte
precursor

CTM
calibration and test
material

CTN
Certified Transcultural
Nurse

CTP
cytidine triphosphate

CTR
cardiothoracic ratio
carpal tunnel release

CTS
carpal tunnel syndrome

CTX
cyclophosphamide
(Cytoxan)

CTZ
chemoreceptor trigger zone
chlorothiazide

Cu
copper (L. cuprum)

cu
cubic
curved

CUC
chronic ulcerative colitis

cu cm
cubic centimeter

CUG
cystourethrogram

Cuj.
L. cujus (of which)

Cuj. Lib.
L. cujus libet (of any you
desire)

cu mm
cubic millimeter

CuO
cupric oxide

CUSA
Cavitron ultrasonic
aspirator

CV
cardiovascular
cell volume
central venous
cerebrovascular
coefficient of variation
color vision
corpuscular volume
cresyl violet

C.V.
conjugata vera (true
conjugate diameter of the
pelvic inlet)
L. cras vespere (tomorrow
evening)

CVA
cardiovascular accident
cerebrovascular accident
costovertebral angle

CVC
central venous catheter

CVD
cardiovascular disease
color vision deviant

CVF
cyclophosphamide,
vincristine, and
5-fluorouracil

CVH
combined ventricular
hypertrophy
common variable
hypogammaglobulinemia

C.V.O.
L. conjugata vera
obstetrica (obstetric
conjugate diameter of
pelvic inlet)

CVOD
cerebrovascular obstructive disease

CVP
cell volume profile
central venous pressure
cyclophosphamide, vincristine, and prednisone

CVPP
cyclophosphamide, vinblastine, procarbazine, and prednisone

CVR
cardiovascular-renal
cerebrovascular resistance

CVRD
cardiovascular renal disease

CVS
cardiovascular surgery
cardiovascular system
chorionic villus sampling
clean voided specimen

CVT
costovertebral (angle) tenderness

CW
chest wall
clockwise
continuous wave

CWDF
cell wall–deficient bacterial forms

CWI
cardiac work index

CWP
childbirth without pain
coal workers' pneumoconiosis

cwt
hundredweight

Cx
cervix
complaints
convex

CXR
chest x-ray

CxR
chest x-ray

Cy
symbol for cyanogen

Cyath.
L. cyathus (a glassful)

CYC
cyclophosphamide

Cyc
cyclophosphamide

cyclic AMP
cyclic adenosine monophosphate

cyclic GMP
cyclic guanosine monophosphate

Cyclo
cyclophosphamide
cyclopropane

Cyd
cytidine

cyl
cylinder
cylindrical lens

Cys
cysteine

Cys-Cys
cystine

cysto
cystoscopic examination

Cyt
cytosine

Cy/TBI
   cyclophosphamide and
      total body irradiation

CyVADIC
   cyclophosphamide,
      vincristine, doxorubicin,
      and dacarbazine

CZI
   crystalline zinc insulin

D

  dalton
  daughter
  daunorubicin
  deciduous (teeth)
  decimal reduction time
  density
  deuterium
  deuteron
  dextro
  dextrose
  died
  diffusing capacity
  diopter
  distal
  divorced
  dorsal vertebrae (D1–D12)
  dose
  duration
  dwarf (colony)
  vitamin D unit

2,4-D

  2,4-dichlorophenoxyacetic
    acid

D.

  L. da (give)
  L. detur (let it be given)
  L. dexter (right)
  L. dosis (dose)

D

  dilution factor

D_5

  dextrose 5% in water

D_{CO}

  diffusing capacity for
    carbon monoxide

D_L

  diffusing capacity of the
    lung

$D_{L_{CO}}$

  diffusing capacity of the
    lung for carbon monoxide

$D_{L_{O2}}$

  diffusing capacity of the
    lung for oxygen

D/3

  distal third

D-

  dextro-

d

  day
  dead
  death
  deci-
  deoxyribose
  died
  diurnal
  divorced

d.

  L. da (give)
  L. detur (let it be given)
  L. dexter (right)
  L. diem (24 hours)
  L. dosis (dose)

d

  density
  diameter

Δ

  change in a component of a
    physical system
  Delta
  diagnosis
  increment

δ

  the heavy chain of IgD
  the δ chain of hemoglobin
  thickness in a biological
    system, as of a layer of
    fluid

DA

  degenerative arthritis
  developmental age
  dietetic assistant

DA *(continued)*
 diphenylchlorarsine
 direct agglutination
 disaggregated
 dopamine
 ductus arteriosus

D/A
 discharge and advise

Da
 dalton

dA
 deoxyadenosine

da
 days

da-
 deka-

(/)da
 (per) day

DAB
 3′3-diaminobenzidine
  hydrochloride
 dimethylaminoazobenzene

DAC
 digital-to-analog converter

DACT
 dactinomycin

Dact
 dactinomycin

DAD
 delayed afterdepolarization
 dispense as directed

DADDS
 diacetyl
  diaminodiphenylsulfone

dADP
 deoxyadenosine
  diphosphate

DAF
 decay acceleration factor

DAGT
 direct antiglobulin test

DAH
 disordered action of heart

DALA
 delta-aminolevulinic acid

DAM
 degraded amyloid
 diacetylmonoxime

dAMP
 deoxyadenosine
  monophosphate
 deoxyadenosine phosphate

D and C
 dilatation and curettage
 dilation and curettage

DANS
 1-dimethylaminoaphtalene-
  5-sulfonic acid

DAO
 diamine oxidase

DAP
 dihydroxyacetone
  phosphate
 direct agglutination
  pregnancy (test)

DAPI
 4′6-diamidino-2-phenylin-
  dole-2HCl

DAPT
 2,4-diamino-5-phenylthia-
  zole
 direct agglutination
  pregnancy test

Dapt
 Daptazole

DAT
 Dental
  Aptitude/Admission Test
 differential agglutination
  titer
 diphtheria antitoxin
 direct antiglobulin test

dAT
    direct agglutination test

dATP
    deoxyadenosine
      triphosphate

DB
    date of birth
    dextran blue
    distobuccal

dB
    decibel

db
    decibel

DBA
    dibenzanthracene

dBA
    decibel, weighted according
      to the A scale

DBC
    dye-binding capacity

DBCL
    dilute blood clot lysis
      (method)

DBCP
    dibromochloropropane

DBI
    development-at-birth index

DBM
    demineralized bone matrix
    dibromomannitol

DBMS
    database management
      system

DBO
    distobucco-occlusal

DBP
    diastolic blood pressure
    distobuccopulpal
    vitamin D-binding protein

DBS
    Denis Browne splint
    despeciated bovine serum

DC
    dendritic cells
    deoxycholate
    diarrhea, constipation
    diphenylarsine cyanide
    direct current
    discharge
    discontinue
    distocervical
    Doctor of Chiropractic

D/C
    discontinued

D & C
    dilatation and curettage
    dilation and curettage

dC
    deoxycytidine

dc
    discontinue

DCA
    deoxycholate-citrate agar
    desoxycorticosterone
      acetate

DCc
    double concave

dCDP
    deoxycytidine diphosphate

DCF
    direct centrifugal flotation

DCG
    disodium cromoglycate

DCH
    Diploma in Child Health

DCHFB
    diclorohexafluorobutane

DCI
    dichloroisoproterenol

DCLS
deoxycholate citrate lactose saccharose

dCMP
deoxycytidine monophosphate
deoxycytidine phosphate

DCOG
Diploma of the College of Obstetricians and Gynaecologists (British)

D colony
dwarf colony

$D_L CO$ SB
Carbon monoxide diffusing capacity (single breath)

DCP
dibasic calcium phosphate

DCT
direct Coombs' test

DCTMA
desoxycorticosterone trimethylacetate

dCTP
deoxycytidine triphosphate

DCTPA
desoxycorticosterone triphenylacetate

DCx
double convex

DD
dependent drainage
died of the disease
differential diagnosis
dry dressing

dd
dideoxynucleoside
dry dressing

d.d.
L. detur ad (let it be given to)

DDAVP
desmopressin

dDAVP
desmopressin

DDBJ
DNA Database of Japan

DDC
diethyldithiocarbamate

ddC
dideoxycytidine

DDD
dense deposit disease
dichlorodiphenyldichloroeth-ane
dihydroxydinaphthyl disulfide
universal (pacemaker code)

o, p-DDD
mitotane

DDI
atrioventricular sequential (pacemaker code)

ddI
dideoxyinosine

DDP
cisplatin (*cis*-dichlorodiammineplati-num II)

Ddp
cisplatin (*cis*-dichlorodiammineplati-num II)

DDS
Doctor of Dental Surgery
diaminodiphenylsulfone
dystrophy-dystocia syndrome

DDSc
Doctor of Dental Science

DDST
Denver Developmental
Screening Test

DDT
chlorophenothane
dichlorodiphenyltrichloroeth-
ane

DDTC
diethyldithiocarbamate

DDVP
dichlorvos

DDX
differential diagnosis

D&E
dilatation and evacuation
dilation and evacuation

DEA
dehydroepiandrosterone
diethanolamine

DEAE
diethylaminoethanol
diethylaminoethyl

DEAE cellulose
diethylaminoethyl
cellulose

DEAE-D
diethylaminoethyl dextran

DEBA
diethylbarbituric acid

Deb. spis.
L. debita spissitudine (of
the proper consistency)

Dec.
L. decanta (pour off)

dec
decompose

Decoct.
L. decoctum (a decoction)

decomp
decompose

decompn
decomposition

DECR
decrease

Decub.
L. decubitus (lying down)

DED
diabetic eye disease

de d. in d.
L. de die in diem (from day
to day)

DEEG
depth
electroencephalogram
depth
electroencephalography
depth electrography

DEF
decayed, extracted, and
filled
defecation
deficiency

def
decayed, extracted, and
filled
defecation
deficiency

ΔEF
ejection fraction response

defic
deficiency

Deg
degeneration
degree

Deglut.
L. deglutiatur (let it be
swallowed)

del
delivery

deliquesc
deliquescent

Dem
  Demerol (meperidine)

Dep.
  L. depuratus (purified)

DeR
  reaction of degeneration

der
  derivative chromosome

deriv
  derivative

DES
  diethylstilbestrol

Des
  diethylstilbestrol

dest.
  L. destilla (distill)
  destillatus (distilled)

destil.
  L. destilla (distill)

DET
  diethyltryptamine

Det.
  L. detur (let it be given)

determn
  determination

Det. in dup., Det. in 2 plo.
  L. detur in duplo (let twice
    as much be given)

D. et s.
  L. detur et signetur (let it
    be given and labeled)

DEV
  duck embryo rabies
    vaccine

DEX
  dexamethasone

Dex
  dexamethasone

DEXA
  dual energy x-ray
    absorptiometry

DF
  decapacitation factor
  decayed and filled
  deficiency factor
  desferrioxamine
  diabetic father
  discriminant function
  dorsiflexion

DF-2
  bacillus

Df
  duodenal fluid

dF
  disseminated foci

df
  decayed and filled
  degrees of freedom
  diabetic father
  dorsiflexion

DFA
  direct fluorescent antibody
  direct fluorescent antibody
    test

DFDT
  difluorodiphenyltrichloroeth-
    ane

DFMO
  difluoromethylornithine

DFO
  deferoxamine

DFOM
  deferoxamine

DFP
  diisopropyl
    fluorophosphate

DFS
  disease-free survival

DFU
  dead fetus in utero
  dideoxyfluorouridine

DG
  deoxyglucose
  diastolic gallop
  diglyceride
  distogingival

dG
  deoxyguanosine

dg
  decigram

dGDP
  deoxyguanosine
  diphosphate

DGGE
  denaturing gradient gel
  electrophoresis

dgm
  decigram

dGMP
  deoxyguanosine
  monophosphate
  deoxyguanosine phosphate

dGTP
  deoxyguanosine
  triphosphate

DH
  delayed hypersensitivity
  diffuse histiocytic
  lymphoma

DHA
  dehydroepiandrosterone
  dihydroxyacetone

Dha
  dihydroalanine

DHAP
  dihydroxyacetone
  phosphate

DHAS
  dehydroepiandrosterone
  sulfate

Dhb
  dehydrobutyrine,
  β-methyl-dehydroalanine

DHE
  dihydroergotamine

DHEA
  dehydroepiandrosterone

DHEAS
  dehydroepiandrosterone
  sulfate

DHEW
  Department of Health,
  Education, and Welfare

DHFR
  dihydrofolate reductase

DHg
  Doctor of Hygiene

DHHS
  Department of Health and
  Human Services

DHIA
  dehydroisoandrosterone

DHL
  diffuse histiocytic
  lymphoma

DHMA
  dihydroxymandelic acid

DHO
  Dhori orthomyxovirus

DHT
  dihydrotachysterol
  dihydrotestosterone

DHy
  Doctor of Hygiene

DI
  diabetes insipidus

DI *(continued)*
　　diagnostic imaging

diag
　　diagnosis
　　diagnostic

diam
　　diameter

DIC
　　diffuse intravascular
　　　coagulation
　　disseminated intravascular
　　　coagulation

dic
　　dicentric

DIE
　　died in Emergency Room

Dieb. alt.
　　L. diebus alternis (on
　　　alternate days)

Dieb. tert.
　　L. diebus tertiis (every
　　　third day)

diff
　　difference
　　differential
　　differential blood count

Dig.
　　digoxin
　　L. digeratur (let it be
　　　digested)

dil.
　　L. dilue (dilute or dissolve)

DILD
　　diffuse infiltrative lung
　　　disease

Diluc.
　　L. diluculo (at daybreak)

dilut.
　　L. dilutus (diluted)

DIM
　　divalent ion metabolism

dim.
　　L. dimidius (one half)

D. in p. aeq.
　　L. divide in partes aequales
　　　(divide into equal parts)

DIP
　　desquamative interstitial
　　　pneumonia
　　desquamative interstitial
　　　pneumonitis
　　diisopropyl phosphate
　　distal interphalangeal
　　　(joint)
　　dual-in-line package

DIPJ
　　distal interphalangeal joint

dir
　　L. directione (directions)

Dir. prop.
　　L. directione propria (with
　　　a proper direction)

disc
　　discontinue

disch
　　discharge

DISH
　　diffuse idiopathic skeletal
　　　hyperostosis

DISI
　　dorsiflexed intercalated
　　　segment instability

Disl
　　dislocation

disp
　　dispense

Dist.
　　L. distilla (distill)

distal/3
　　distal third

distln
    distillation

DIT
    diiodotyrosine

Div.
    L. divide (divide)

div
    division

DJD
    degenerative joint disease

DK
    decay
    diseased kidney

DKA
    diabetic ketoacidosis

DKB
    deep knee bends

DL
    danger list
    difference limen
    diffusing capacity of the
      lung
    distolingual
    Donath-Landsteiner (test)
    doxorubicin and lomustine
    racemic

DL-
    racemic

dL
    deciliter

dl
    deciliter

dl-
    racemic

DLA
    distolabial

D-L Ab
    Donath-Landsteiner
      antibody

DLAI
    distolabioincisal

DLCO
    diffusing capacity of the
      lung for carbon monoxide

$D_{L_{CO}}RB$
    diffusing capacity of the
      lung, rebreathing
      methods

$D_{L_{CO}}SB$
    diffusing capacity of the
      lung, single breath

$D_{L_{CO}}SS$
    diffusing capacity of the
      lung, steady state

DLE
    discoid lupus
      erythematosus
    disseminated lupus
      erythematosus

DLI
    distolinguoincisal

DLO
    distolinguo-occlusal

DLP
    distolinguopulpal

DM
    diabetes mellitus
    diabetic mother
    diastolic murmur
    diffuse mixed
      histiocytic-lymphocytic
      lymphoma
    diphenylamine-arsine
      chloride
    dopamine

dM
    decimorgan

dm
    decimeter

DMA
dimethoxyamphetamine
dimethyladenosine
direct memory access

DMAB
dimethylbenzanthracene

DMARD
disease modifying
antirheumatic drug

DMAT
Disaster Medical
Assistance Team

DMBA
7,12-dimethylbenz[a]anthra-
cene

DMC
p,p′-dichlorodiphenyl
methyl carbinol

DMCT
demeclocycline
hydrochloride
demethylchlortetracycline

DMD
Doctor of Dental Medicine
Duchenne's muscular
dystrophy

DME
dimethyl ether (of
D-TUBOCURARINE)

DMF
decayed, missing, filled
(teeth)
dimethylformamide

DMFS
decayed, missing, and filled
surfaces

DMFT
DMF used with the tooth
as the unit of
measurement

DMI
diaphragmatic myocardial
infarction

DML
diffuse mixed
histiocytic-lymphocytic
lymphoma

DMM
dimethylmyleran

DMN
dimethylnitrosamine

DMO
dimethadione

DMPA
depomedroxyprogesterone
acetate

DMPE
3,4-dimethoxyphenylethyl-
amine

DMPP
dimethylphenylpipera-
zinium

DMRD
Diploma in Medical
Radio-Diagnosis (British)

DMRT
Diploma in Medical
Radio-Therapy (British)

DMS
dimethyl sulfoxide

DMSO
dimethyl sulfoxide

DMT
dimethyltryptamine

DN
dextrose-nitrogen (ratio)
dibucaine number

Dn.
dekanem

dn.
    decinem

DNA
    deoxyribonucleic acid
    did not answer (or appear)

DNase
    deoxyribonuclease

DNB
    Dictionary of National
        Biography
    dinitrobenzene
    Diplomate of the National
        Board (of Medical
        Examiners)

DNC
    dinitrocarbanilide

DNCB
    dinitrochlorobenzene

DND
    died a natural death

DNFB
    dinitrofluorobenzene

DNJ
    deoxynojirimycin

DNOC
    dinitro-o-cresol

DNP
    deoxyribonucleoprotein
    2,4-dinitrophenol

Dnp
    2,4-dinitrophenol
    deoxyribonucleoprotein

DNPH
    dinitrophenylhydrazine

DNPM
    dinitrophenylmorphine

DNR
    daunorubicin
    do not resuscitate

Dnr
    daunorubicin

DNS
    dansyl
    Doctor of Nursing Science

Dns
    dansyl

DNSc.
    Doctor of Nursing Science

d_5NS
    dextrose 5% in normal
        saline

D5NS
    5% dextrose in normal
        saline

D5/NS
    5% dextrose in normal
        saline

D5%/NS
    5% dextrose in normal
        saline

D_5NSS
    5% dextrose in normal
        saline solution

DNT
    did not test

DO
    diamine oxidase
    disto-occlusal
    Doctor of Osteopathy
    doctor's orders

DOA
    date of admission
    dead on arrival

DOB
    date of birth

DOC
    deoxycholate
    11-deoxycorticosterone
    died of other causes

DOCA
    deoxycorticosterone
       acetate

DOCS
    deoxycorticoids

DOD
    date of death
    Department of Defense
    drug overdose

DOE
    date of examination
    Department of Energy
    dyspnea on exercise
    dyspnea on exertion

DOM
    deaminated -*O*-methyl
       metabolite
    2,5-dimethoxy-4-methylam-
       phetamine

DOMA
    dihydroxymandelic acid

DON
    Determination of Need
    diazo-oxonorleucine
    Director of Nursing

Donec alv. sol. fuerit
    L. donec alvus soluta fuerit
       (until the bowels are
       opened)

Dopa
    dihydroxyphenylalanine

DOPAC
    dihydroxyphenylacetic acid

DOXO
    doxorubicin

Doxo
    doxorubicin

DP
    dementia praecox
    diastolic pressure
    distal phalanx
    distopulpal

DP *(continued)*
    Doctor of Pharmacy
    Doctor of Podiatry
    dorsalis pedis

D.P.
    L. directione propria (with
       proper direction)

dp
    dorsalis pedis
    degree of polymerization

DPA
    dipropylacetate
    dual photon
       absorptiometry

DPC
    delayed primary closure
    distal palmar crease

DPD
    diffuse pulmonary disease

DPDL
    diffuse poorly
       differentiated
       lymphocytic lymphoma

dpdt
    double-pole double-throw
       (switch)

DPG
    2,3-diphosphoglycerate
    displacement placentogram

2,3-DPG
    2,3-diphosphoglycerate

DPGM
    diphosphoglyceromutase

DPGP
    diphosphoglycerate
       phosphatase

DPH
    diphenylhydantoin
    Diploma in Public Health

DPL
    distopulpolingual

DPM
Diploma in Psychological
Medicine
disintegrations per minute
Doctor of Podiatric
Medicine

dpm
disintegrations per minute

DPN
diphosphopyridine
nucleotide

DPN$^+$
oxidized diphosphopyridine
nucleotide

DPNase
NAD$^+$nucleosidase

DPNH
reduced form of
diphosphopyridine
nucleotide (now described
as the reduced form of
nicotinamide-adenine
dinucleotide and
symbolized NADH)

DPP
dimethoxyphenyl penicillin

DPS
dimethylpolysiloxane

dpst
double-pole single-throw
(switch)

DPT
Demerol Phenergan
Thorazine
diphtheria-pertussis-tetanus-
(vaccine)
dipropyltryptamine

DPTA
diethylenetriamine
pentaacetic acid

DQ
developmental quotient

DR
delivery room
diabetic retinopathy
diagnostic radiology
reaction of degeneration

Dr
doctor

dr
dram

DREZ
dorsal root entry zone

DRF
dose-reduction factor

DRG
diagnosis-related group

DRI
discharge readiness
inventory

dRNA
DNA-like RNA

DRNR
(certificate in) diagnostic
radiology with special
competence in nuclear
radiology

DrPH
Doctor of Public Health

DRTA
distal renal tubular
acidosis

DS
defined substrate
dehydroepiandrosterone
sulfate
dextrose-saline
Doctor of Science
Down syndrome

D/S
(5%) dextrose in (0.9%)
saline (sodium chloride)

ds
    double stranded

DSA
    digital subtraction
        angiography

DSAP
    disseminated superficial
        actinic porokeratosis

DSC
    differential scanning
        colorimetry
    disodium cromoglycate
    Doctor of Surgical
        Chiropody

DSc
    Doctor of Science

DSCG
    disodium cromoglycate

DSD
    dry sterile dressing

dsDNA
    double-stranded DNA

dsg
    dressing

DSM
    dextrose solution mixture

DSM-III-R
    Diagnostic and Statistical
        Manual of Mental
        Disorders

D-spine
    dorsal spine

dsRNA
    double-stranded RNA

DST
    dexamethasone
        suppression test
    donor specific transfusion

D-state
    REM sleep

DT
    delirium tremens
    dye test

Dt
    duration tetany

dT
    deoxythymidine

DTA
    differential thermal
        analysis

DTAA
    di-tryptophan animal and
        acetaldehyde

DTBC
    tubocurarine

D.T.D.
    L. datur talis dosis (give of
        such a dose)

dTDP
    deoxythymidine
        diphosphate

DTF
    detector transfer function

DTH
    delayed type
        hypersensitivity

Δ9 THC
    delta-9-tetrahydrocannabin-
        ol

dThd
    thymidine

DTIC
    dacarbazine

Dtic
    dacarbazine
        (dimethyltriazenoimid-
        azole carboxamide)

DTM
    dermatophyte test medium

dTMP
    deoxythymidine
        monophosphate

DTN
    diphtheria toxin normal

DTNB
    dithiobisnitrobenzoic acid

DTP
    diphtheria, tetanus, and
        pertussis
    distal tingling on
        percussion

DTPA
    pentetic acid

DTPA In 111
    the diethylenetetramine-
        pentaacetic acid chelate
        of indium 111

DTPA In 113m
    the diethylenetetramine-
        pentaacetic acid chelate
        of indium 113m

DTPA Tc 99m
    the diethylenetetramine-
        pentaacetic acid chelate
        of technetium 99m

DTR
    deep tendon reflex
    registered dietetic
        technician

Dts
    delirium tremens

DTT
    diphtheria tetanus toxoid
    dithiothreitol

dTTP
    deoxythymidine
        triphosphate

DTV
    due to void

DTX
    dimethyl triazino imidazol
        carboxamide

DTZ
    diatrizoate

DU
    diagnosis undetermined
    diffuse undifferentiated
        lymphoma
    duodenal ulcer

dU
    deoxyuridine

du
    dial unit

DUB
    dysfunctional uterine
        bleeding

dUMP
    deoxyuridine
        monophosphate
    deoxyuridine phosphate

duod
    duodenum

Dur. dolor.
    L. durante dolore (while
        the pain lasts)

dUTP
    deoxyuridine triphosphate

DV
    dependent variable
    dilute volume

D&V
    diarrhea and vomiting

dv
    double vibrations

DVA
    distance visual acuity

DVD
    dissociated vertical
        divergence (or deviation)

DVI
    atrioventricular sequential
        (pacemaker code)

DVIU
    direct vision internal
        urethrotomy

DVM
    digital voltmeter
    Doctor of Veterinary
        Medicine

DVMS
    Doctor of Veterinary
        Medicine and Surgery

DVP-Asp
    daunorubicin, vincristine,
        prednisone and
        asparaginase

DVS
    Doctor of Veterinary
        Science
    Doctor of Veterinary
        Surgery

DVSA
    digital venous subtraction
        angiography

DVT
    deep venous thrombosis

DW
    dextrose in water
    distilled water

D/W
    dextrose in water

D5W
    5% dextrose in water

D$_5$W
    5% dextrose in water

D5&W
    5% dextrose in water

DWDL
    diffuse well-differentiated
        lymphocytic leukemia
    diffuse well-differentiated
        lymphocytic lymphoma

dwt
    pennyweight

DX
    dextran
    diagnosis

Dx
    diagnosis

DXM
    dexamethasone

DXRT
    deep x-ray therapy

DXT
    deep x-ray therapy

Dy
    dysprosium

dyn
    dyne

DZ
    dizygotic
    dizziness
    dizzy

E

cortisone (compound E)
electric charge
electron
emmetropia
enzyme
epinephrine
exa-
extraction fraction
eye

4E

four plus edema

E

elastance
electromotive force
energy
expectancy
illumination
electric intensity
Entamoeba
Escherichia
redox potential

E_1

estrone

E_2

estradiol

E_3

estriol

E_4

estetrol

$E_0 +$

oxidation-reduction
potential

E^0

oxidation-reduction
potential

E_M

molar extinction coefficient

E_O

electroaffinity

E_h

redox potential

E°

standard reduction
potential

e

electron
erythrocyte
the base of natural
logarithms
(approximately
2.7182818285)

e

elementary unit of electric
charge

e^+

positron

e^-

electron
the heavy chain of IgE
the ϵ chain of hemoglobin
molar absorptivity

η

absolute viscosity
apparent (or dynamic)
velocity

EA

early antigen
educational age
erythrocyte antibody
ethacrynic acid

EAA

excitatory amino acid

EAC

Ehrlich ascites carcinoma
erythrocyte antibody and
complement
external auditory canal

EACA
epsilon-aminocaproic acid

EACH
Essential Access
Community Hospital

ε-Acp
ε-aminocaproic acid

EAD
early afterdepolarization

ead.
L. eadem (the same)

EAE
experimental allergic
encephalomyelitis

EAEC
enteroadherent
(*Escherichia coli*)

EAHF
eczema, asthma, hay fever

EAHLG
equine antihuman
lymphoblast globulin

EAHLS
equine antihuman
lymphoblast serum

EAM
external auditory meatus

EAN
experimental allergic
neuritis

EAP
epiallopregnanolone
etoposide, doxorubicin, and
cisplatin

Ea. R.
Ger. Entartungs-Reaktion
(reaction of degeneration)

EB
elementary body
epidermolysis bullosa

EB *(continued)*
Epstein-Barr
estradiol benzoate

EBF
erythroblastosis fetalis

EBI
emetine bismuth iodide

EBL
estimated blood loss

EBM
expressed breast milk

EBNA
Epstein-Barr nuclear
antigen (test)

EBV
Epstein-Barr virus

EC
electrochemical
electron capture
enteric coated
Enzyme Commission
Escherichia coli
excitation-contraction
experimental control
extracellular
eyes closed

ECA
ethacrynic acid

ECBO virus
enteric cytopathogenic
bovine orphan virus

ECBV
effective circulating blood
volume

ECC
extracorporeal circulation

ECD
electron capture detectors

ECDO virus
enteric cytopathogenic dog
orphan virus

ECF
    effective capillary flow
    eosinophil chemotactic
      factor
    extended care facility
    extracellular fluid

ECF-A
    eosinophil chemotactic
      factor of anaphylaxis

ECFMG
    Educational Council for
      Foreign Medical
      Graduates

ECFV
    extracellular fluid volume

ECG
    electrocardiogram
    electrogastrography

ECHO
    echocardiogram
    enteric cytopathogenic
      human orphan (virus)

ECI
    electrocerebral inactivity
    extracorporeal irradiation
      of blood

ECIB
    extracorporeal irradiation
      of blood

ECIL
    extracorporeal irradiation
      of lymph

ECL
    emitter-coupled logic

ECLT
    euglobulin clot lysis time

ECM
    erythema chronicum
      migrans
    extracellular material

ECMO
    extracorporeal membrane
      oxygenation

ECMO virus
    enteric cytopathogenic
      monkey orphan virus

ECOG
    Eastern Cooperative
      Oncology Group

ECoG
    electrocorticogram
    electrocorticography

E. coli
    Escherichia coli

econ
    economic
    economics

ECRB
    extensor carpi radialis
      brevis

ECRL
    extensor carpi radialis
      longus

ECS
    electrocerebral silence
    electroconvulsive shock

ECSO virus
    enteric cytopathogenic
      swine orphan virus

ECT
    electroconvulsive therapy
    euglobulin clot test

ECU
    extensor carpi ulnaris

ECV
    extracellular volume

ECW
    extracellular water

ED
    effective dose

ED *(continued)*
 elbow disarticulation
 Ehlers-Danlos syndrome
 Emergency Department
 epidural
 epileptiform discharge
 erythema dose
 extensive disease

ED$_{50}$
 median effective dose

ed
 edema
 edition

EDA
 ethylenediamine

EDB
 ethylene dibromide

EDC
 estimated date of
   confinement
 expected date of
   confinement
 extensor digitorum
   communis

EDD
 estimated date of delivery
 expected date of delivery

EDF
 eosinophil differentiation
   factor

EDIM
 epidemic diarrhea of infant
   mice

EDL
 extensor digitorum longus

EDP
 end diastolic pressure

EDQ
 extensor digiti quinti

EDR
 effective direct radiation

EDR *(continued)*
 electrodermal response

EDRF
 endothelium-derived
   relaxing factor

EDS
 Ehlers-Danlos syndrome

EDS '76
 egg-drop syndrome

Ed(s)
 editor(s)

EDTA
 edetic acid
 ethylenediaminetetraacetic
   acid

educ
 education

EDV
 end-diastolic volume

EDVI
 end-diastolic volume index

EDX
 electrodiagnosis
 energy-dispersive x-ray
   analysis

EE
 end to end
 equine encephalitis
 eye and ear

EEA
 electroencephalic
   audiometry

EEC
 enteropathogenic
   Escherichia coli

EEE
 eastern equine
   encephalomyelitis (virus)

EEE virus
 eastern equine
   encephalomyelitis virus

EEG
electroencephalogram
electroencephalography

EEME
ethinylestradiol methyl
ether

EENT
eye-ear-nose-throat

EER
electroencephalic response

EERP
extended endocardial
resection procedure

EESHRTS
Entrance Examination for
Schools of Health-Related
Technologies

EF
ectopic focus
ejection fraction
encephalitogenic factor
extended field (irradiation)

EFA
essential fatty acids

EFC
endogenous fecal calcium

EFE
endocardial fibroelastosis

EFV
extracellular fluid volume

EFVC
expiratory flow-volume
curve

EG
esophagogastrectomy

e.g.
L. exempli gratia (for
example)

EGB
eosinophilic granuloma of
bone

EGD
esophagogastroduodenos-
copy

EGF
epidermal growth factor

EGF-R
epidermal growth factor
receptor

EGG
electrogastrogram

EGL
eosinophilic granuloma of
the lung

EGM
electrogram

EGOT
erythrocyte glutamic
oxaloacetic transaminase

EH
enlarged heart
essential hypertension

EHBF
estimated hepatic blood
flow
extrahepatic blood flow

EHC
enterohepatic circulation
essential
hypercholesterolemia

EHD
epizootic hemorrhagic
disease

EHDP
ethane-1-hydroxy-1,1-dipho-
sphonate

EHEC
enterohemorrhagic
(*Escherichia coli*)

EHF
exophthalmos-hyperthyroid-factor

EHL
endogenous hyperlipidemia
extensor hallucis longus

EHO
extrahepatic obstruction

EHP
excessive heat production

EI
enzyme inhibitor
eosinophilic index

E/I
expiration-inspiration ratio

EIA
electroimmunoassay
enzyme immunoassay

EID
electroimmunodiffusion
emergency infusion device

EIEC
enteroinvasive *Escherichia coli*

EIP
extensor indicis proprius

eIPV
enhanced potency inactivated poliovirus vaccine

EIT
erythrocyte iron turnover

EJ
elbow jerk

EJN
external jugular vein

Ejusd.
L. ejusdem (of the same)

EK
erythrokinase

EKC
epidemic keratoconjunctivitis

EKG
electrocardiogram

EKY
electrokymogram

ELAM
endothelial cell leukocyte adhesion molecule

Elecs
electrolytes

ELISA
enzyme-linked immunosorbent assay

Elix
elixir

ELPS
excessive lateral pressure syndrome

ELT
euglobulin lysis time

EM
ejection murmur
electron microscope
electron microscopic
electron microscopy
erythrocyte mass

Em
emmetropia

EMA-CO
etoposide, methotrexate, dactinomycin, cyclophosphamide, vincristine

EMB
eosin-methylene blue
ethambutol
ethambutol-Myambutol

EMBL
European Molecular
Biology Laboratory

EMC
electron microscopy
encephalomyocarditis
(virus)

EMC virus
encephalomyocarditis virus

EMF
electromagnetic flowmeter
electromotive force
endomyocardial fibrosis
erythrocyte maturation
factor

EMG
electromyelogram
electromyogram
electromyography
exophthalmos,
macroglossia, gigantism

EMI
electromagnetic
interference

EMIC
emergency maternity and
infant care

EMIT
enzyme-multiplied
immunoassay technique

Emp.
L. emplastrum (a plaster)

e.m.p.
L. ex modo praescripto (in
the manner prescribed)

EMS
Emergency Medical
Service (British)

EMSU
early morning specimen of
urine

EMT
emergency medical
technician

emu
electromagnetic unit

emul.
L. emulsum (emulsion)

EN
erythema nodosum

en
ethylenediamine

ENA
Emergency Nurses
Association
extractable nuclear
antigens

end
endoreduplication

ENE
ethylnorepinephrine

ENG
electronystagmography

ENL
erythema nodosum
leprosum

ENS
(ethylnorsuprarenin)

ENT
ear, nose, and throat

environ
environment
environmental

EO
eosinophil
eosinophilia
ethylene oxide
eyes open

EOA
esophageal obturator

EOG
electro-oculogram
electro-olfactogram

EOM
extraocular movement
extraocular muscles

EORTC
European Organization for
Research in Cancer
Therapy

Eos
eosinophils

eos
eosinophil

EOT
effective oxygen transport

EP
ectopic pregnancy
electrophoresis
endogenous pyrogen
erythrocyte protoporphyrin
evoked potential

Ep
epilepsy

EPA
eicosapentaenoic acid
Environmental Protection
Agency

EPB
extensor pollicis brevis

EPC
epilepsia partialis continua

EPEC
enteropathogenic
Escherichia coli

EPF
exophthalmos-producing
factor

EPI
epinephrine
Expanded Program of
Immunization

epith
epithelial

EPL
extensor pollicis longus

EPM
electronic pacemaker

EPO
erythropoietin

EPP
end-plate potential
equal pressure point
erythropoietic
protoporphyria

EPR
electron paramagnetic
resonance
electrophrenic respiration
estradiol production rate

EPS
electrophysiologic study
exophthalmos-producing
substance
extrapyramidal signs
extrapyramidal symptoms

EPSP
excitatory postsynaptic
potential

EPTS
existed prior to service

EQ
educational quotient

eq
equation
equivalent

equil
equilibrium

equiv
equivalent

ER
ejection rate
emergency room

ER *(continued)*
    endoplasmic reticulum
    estrogen receptors
    evoked response
    external resistance

Er
    erbium

er
    emergency room
    endoplasmic reticulum
    estrogen receptors

ERA
    electric response
      audiometry
    evoked response
      audiometry

ERBF
    effective renal blood flow

ERC
    erythropoietin-responsive
      cell

Erc
    erythrocyte

ERCP
    endoscopic retrograde
      cholangiopancreato-
      graphy

Ercs
    erythrocytes
    external rotation in
      extension

ERF
    external rotation in flexion

ERG
    electroretinogram

ER-ICA
    estrogen receptor-immuno-
      cytochemical assay

ERP
    effective refractory period
    endocardial resection
      procedure

ERP *(continued)*
    equine rhinopneumonitis

ERPF
    effective renal plasma flow

ERT
    estrogen replacement
      therapy

ERV
    expiratory reserve volume

ES
    emission spectroscopy
    end-to-side

Es
    einsteinium

ESB
    electrical stimulation to
      brain

Esch
    Escherichia

ESEP
    extreme somatosensory
      evoked potential

ESF
    erythropoietic stimulating
      factor

ESIN
    elastic stable
      intramedullary nailing

ESL
    end-systolic length

ESM
    ejection systolic murmur

eso
    esophagoscopy
    esophagus

ESP
    end systolic pressure
    eosinophil stimulation
      promoter
    extrasensory perception

esp
especially

ESR
erythrocyte sedimentation rate

esr
electron spin resistance

ESRD
end stage renal disease

ESS
erythrocyte-sensitizing substance

ess
essential

EST
electroshock therapy

e.s.u.
electrostatic unit

ESV
end-systolic volume

ESVI
end-systolic volume index

ESWL
extracorporeal shock wave lithotripsy

ET
effective temperature
ejection time
endotracheal
etiology
eustachian tube

Et
ethyl group

ETA
ethionamide

et. al.
L. et alii (and others)

etc.
L. et cetera (and so forth)

ETEC
enterotoxic *Escherichia coli*
enterotoxigenic *Escherichia coli*

ETF
electron transfer flavoprotein
eustachian tube function

ETH
elixir terpin hydrate

ETH/C
elixir terpin hydrate with codeine

ETHcC
elixir terpin hydrate with codeine

etiol
etiology

ETKM
every test known to man

ETKTM
every test known to man

ETM
erythromycin

Etn
ethanolamine

ET-NANB
enterically transmitted non-A, non-B hepatitis

Et$_2$O
ether

ETOH
ethanol

EtOH
ethanol

ETOP
etoposide

Etop
    etoposide

ETOX
    ethylene oxide

ETP
    eustachian tube pressure

ETT
    exercise tolerance test
    extrathyroidal thyroxine

ETU
    emergency and trauma
        unit

EU
    Ehrlich unit
    endotoxin unit
    enzyme unit

Eu
    europium

EUA
    examination under
        anesthesia

EV
    epidermodysplasia
        verruciformis
    extravascular

eV
    electron volt

ev
    electron volt

EVA
    etoposide, vincristine, and
        doxorubicin

evac
    evacuated
    evacuation

eval
    evaluate
    evaluation

EVAP
    etoposide, vinblastine,
        cytarabine, and cisplatin

evapn
    evaporation

EVM
    electronic voltmeter

EW
    emergency ward

ew
    elsewhere

EWB
    estrogen withdrawal
        bleeding

EWL
    egg-white lysozyme

Ex
    exercise

ex
    excision
    exophthalmos

exam
    examination
    examiner

EXBF
    exercise hyperemia blood
        flow

exc
    excision

exec
    executive

Exhib.
    L. exhibeatur (let it be
        given)

exp
    exploration
    expose
    exposure

exper
    experimental

expir
    expiration

exp lap
    exploratory laparotomy
expt
    experiment
ext.
    exterior
    external
    extract

extern.
    externally
extr
    extremity
ext rot
    external rotation

F
- Fahrenheit
- farad
- father
- feces
- female
- fertility (plasmid)
- finger
- fluorine
- foramen
- force
- formula
- French (scale)
- hydrocortisone
- visual field

F.
- L. fiat (let it be done)

F-12
- Freon 12

F
- faraday
- *Filaria*
- force
- *fusiformis*
- gilbert
- luminous flux

F_1
- first filial generation

F_2
- second filial generation

°F
- degree Fahrenheit

f
- fasting
- femto-
- focal length

f
- frequency
- furanose

FA
- false aneurysm
- fatty acid
- femoral artery
- fluorescent antibody
- folic acid
- free acid
- forearm

fa
- father

FAAN
- Fellow of the American Academy of Nursing

FAA sol
- formalin, acetic, alcohol solution

FAB
- formalin ammonium bromide
- French-American-British classification system used for certain leukemias
- functional arm brace

Fab
- fragment, antigen-binding

$F(ab)_2$
- symbol for a fragment of an immunoglobulin G molecule

FABER
- flexion in abduction and external rotation

FAC
- fluorouracil, doxorubicin, cyclophosphamide

FACA
- Fellow of the American College of Anesthesiologists

FACD
Fellow of the American College of Dentists

FACOG
Fellow of the American College of Obstetricians and Gynecologists

FACP
Fellow of the American College of Physicians

FACR
Fellow of the American College of Radiologists

FACS
Fellow of the American College of Surgeons
fluorescence-activated cell sorter

FACSM
Fellow of the American College of Sports Medicine

FAD
flavin adenine dinucleotide

FADF
fluorescent antibody darkfield

FADIR
flexion in adduction and internal rotation

Fahr
Fahrenheit

FAI
functional aerobic impairment

FAM
fluorouracil, doxorubicin, mitomycin C

FAMA
fluorescent antibody to membrane antigen

FAMe
5-fluorouracil, doxorubicin, and semustine

FAN
fuchsin, amido black, and naphthol yellow

FANA
fluorescent antinuclear antibody

FAO
Food and Agriculture Organization

FAOTA
Fellow, American Occupational Therapy Association

FAP
familial adenomatous polyposis
fluorouracil, doxorubicin, cisplatin

FAPHA
Fellow of the American Public Health Association

fasc.
L. fasciculus (bundle)

FASEB
Federation of American Societies for Experimental Biology

FAT
fluorescent antibody test
5-fluorouracil, doxorubicin, and trazinate

FAV
feline ataxia virus

FB
finger breadth
foreign body

FBD
functional bowel disorder

FBE
full blood examination

FBF
forearm blood flow

FBP
femoral blood pressure
fibrinogen breakdown
products

FBS
fasting blood sugar
fetal bovine serum

FC
finger clubbing

Fc
fragment, crystallizable

Fc
a fragment produced in
minute quantities by
papain digestion of
immunoglobulin G
molecules

FCA
ferritin-conjugated
antibodies
Freund's complete
adjuvant

FCAP
Fellow of the College of
American Pathologists

FCC
Federal Communications
Commission
follicular center cells

FCCP
Fellow of the American
College of Chest
Physicians

fCi
femtocurie

FCP(SA)
Fellow of the College of
Physicians of South
Africa

FCR
flexor carpi radialis

FCU
flexor carpi ulnaris

FD
fatal dose
focal distance
forceps delivery

FD_{50}
median fatal dose

Fd
ferredoxin

FDA
Food and Drug
Administration
fronto-dextra anterior
(right frontoanterior)

FD&C
Food, Drug, and Cosmetic
(Act)

FD&C Red No. 2
amaranth

FD&C Red No. 3
erythrosine sodium

FDG
fluorodeoxyglucose

FDI
Fédération Dentaire
Internationale

FDL
flexor digitorum longus

FDNB
fluoro-2,4-dinitrobenzene

FDP
fibrin degradation products
flexor digitorum profundus

FDP *(continued)*
 fronto-dextra posterior
  (right frontoposterior)
 fructose 1,6-diphosphate

FDQB
 flexor digiti quinti brevis

FDS
 flexor digitorum sublimis
 flexor digitorum
  superficialis

FDT
 fronto-dextra transversa
  (right frontotransverse)

F-dUMP
 5-fluorodeoxyuridine
  monophosphate

Fe
 iron

Fe$_{NA}$
 excreted fraction of filtered
  sodium
 fibrinogen degradation
  products

Feb. dur.
 L. febre durante (while the
  fever lasts)

FEC
 free erythrocyte
  coproporphyrin

FECG
 fetal electrocardiogram

FECP
 free erythrocyte
  coproporphyria

FECV
 functional extracellular
  fluid volume

FEF
 forced expiratory flow

FEKG
 fetal electrocardiogram

FEL
 familial erythrophagocytic
  lymphohistiocytosis

FeLV
 feline leukemia virus

FEM
 femoral
 femur

fem
 femoral
 femur

Fem. intern.
 L. femoribus internus (at
  the inner side of the
  thighs)

FEP
 free erythrocyte
  porphyrins
 free erythrocyte
  protoporphyrin

FEPP
 free erythrocyte
  protoporphyrin

Ferv.
 L. fervens (boiling)

FES
 flame emission
  spectrophotometry
 forced expiratory
  spirogram
 functional electrical
  stimulation

FeSO$_4$
 ferrous sulfate

FET
 forced expiratory time

FETS
 forced expiratory time, in
  seconds

FEV
 forced expiratory volume

FEV$_1$
> 1-sec forced expiratory
> volume

FF
> fat free
> fecal frequency
> filtration fraction
> finger to finger
> flat feet
> force fluids
> foster father
> further flexion

ff
> following

FFA
> free fatty acids

FFC
> fixed flexion contracture
> free from chlorine

FFDW
> fat-free dry weight

FFM
> fat-free mass

FFP
> fresh frozen plasma

FFPS
> Fellow of the Faculty of
> Physicians and Surgeons
> (Glasgow)

FFR
> freedom from relapse

FFT
> flicker fusion threshold

FFWW
> fat-free wet weight

FG
> fibrinogen

FGD
> fatal granulomatous
> disease

FH
> familial
> hypercholesterolemia
> family history
> fetal head
> fetal heart

F.h.
> L. fiat haustus (let a
> draught be made)

FHH
> familial hypocalciuric
> hypercalcemia

FHNH
> fetal heart not heard

FHR
> fetal heart rate

FHS
> fetal heart sound

FHT
> fetal heart
> fetal heart tone

FI
> fever caused by infection
> fibrinogen
> fibula, complete
> (congenital absence of
> limb)
> flame ionization
> forced inspiration

fi
> fibula, incomplete
> (congenital absence of
> limb)

FIA
> fluoroimmunoassay
> Freud's incomplete
> adjuvant

FIAT
> Field Information Agency,
> Technical

fib
> fibrillation

fib *(continued)*
　　fibrinogen

FIC
　　Fellowship of the Institute
　　　of Chemistry

FICD
　　Fellow of the International
　　　College of Dentists

FICS
　　Fellow of the International
　　　College of Surgeons

FID
　　flame ionization detector

FIF
　　forced inspiratory flow

FIGLU
　　formiminoglutamic acid

FIGO
　　International Federation of
　　　Gynecology and
　　　Obstetrics

FILT
　　filter

FIO$_2$
　　fractional inspired oxygen

FIPV
　　infectious peritonitis virus

fist
　　fistula

FITC
　　fluorescein isothiocyanate

FJN
　　familial juvenile
　　　nephrophthisis

FJP
　　familial juvenile polyposis

FJROM
　　full joint range of motion

FKQCP
　　Fellow of the King and
　　　Queen's College of
　　　Physicians (of Ireland)

FL
　　filtered load

Fl.
　　fluid

fL
　　femtoliter

fl
　　flourished (in historical
　　　dates)
　　fluid

FLA
　　fronto-laeva anterior (left
　　　frontoanterior)

F.l.a.
　　L. fiat lege artis (let it be
　　　done according to rule)

fld
　　fluid

fl dr
　　fluid dram

FLEX
　　Federation licensing
　　　examination

FLK
　　funny looking kid

Flor.
　　L. flores (flowers)

fl oz
　　fluidounce

FLP
　　fronto-laeva posterior (left
　　　frontoposterior)

FLS
　　Fellow of the Linnean
　　　Society

FLS *(continued)*
    fibrous long-spacing
        (collagen)

FLSA
    follicular lymphosarcoma

FLT
    fronto-laeva transversa
        (left frontotransverse)

fluor.
    fluorometry

FM
    fine motor
    flowmeter

F.M.
    L. fiat mistura (make a
        mixture)

Fm
    fermium

fm
    femtometer

FMC
    Foundation for Medical
        Care

FMD
    foot-and-mouth disease

FME
    full mouth extraction

FMF
    familial Mediterranean
        fever
    fetal movement felt

FMG
    foreign medical graduate

FMN
    flavin mononucleotide
        (riboflavin 5-phosphate)

Fmoc
    9-fluorenylmethoxycar-
        bonyl

fmol
    femtomole

FMP
    first menstrual period

FMS
    fat-mobilizing substance
    financial management
        system
    full mouth series

FN
    false negative
    finger to nose

FNH
    focal nodular hyperplasia

FNS
    functional neuromuscular
        stimulation

FNTC
    fine needle transhepatic
        cholangiography

FO
    foramen ovate
    fronto-occipital

Fo
    forearm
    forearm amputation

FOAVF
    failure of all vital forces

FOB
    fecal occult blood
    feet out of bed

FOD
    free of disease

Fol.
    L. folia (leaves)

FONAR
    Focusing Magnetic Nuclear
        Magnetic Resonance

FORTRAN
formula translation (a computer language)

found
foundation

FP
false positive
family practice
flat plate
flavin phosphate
flavoprotein
freezing point
frontoparietal
frozen plasma

F-P
femoral-popliteal

F.p.
L. fiat potio (let a potion be made)
freezing point

fp
foot-pound
freezing point

FPA
fluorophenylalanine

FPB
femoropopliteal bypass
flexor pollicis brevis

FPC
familial polyposis coli
fish protein concentrate

FPG
fasting plasma glucose

FPIA
fluorescence polarization immunoassay

F.pil.
L. fiant pilulae (let pills be made)

FPL
flexor pollicis longus

FPM
filter paper microscopic (test)

FPS
foot-pound-second

fps
foot-pound-second

FR
family report
Fisher-Race (notation)
flocculation reaction
flow rate

F&R
force and rhythm (pulse)

Fr
francium
French scale

Fract
fracture

Fract. dos.
L. fracta dosi (in divided doses)

frag
fragility

FRC
frozen red cells
functional reserve capacity
functional residual capacity

FRCP
Fellow of the Royal College of Physicians

FRCP(C)
Fellow of the Royal College of Physicians of Canada
Fellow of the Royal College of Physicians of Edinburgh

FRCP(Glasg)
    Fellow of the Royal College
    of Physicians and
    Surgeons of Glasgow qua
    Physician

FRCPI
    Fellow of the Royal College
    of Physicians in Ireland

FRCS
    Fellow of the Royal College
    of Surgeons

FRCS(C)
    Fellow of the Royal College
    of Surgeons of Canada

FRCSE
    Fellow of the Royal College
    of Surgeons of Edinburgh

FRCS(Glasg)
    Fellow of the Royal College
    of Physicians and
    Surgeons of Glasgow qua
    Surgeon

FRCSI
    Fellow of the Royal College
    of Surgeons in Ireland

FRCVS
    Fellow of the Royal College
    of Veterinary Surgeons

freq
    frequent

FRF
    follicle-stimulating
    hormone releasing factor

FRFPS
    Fellow of the Royal
    Faculty of Physicians and
    Surgeons

FRFPSG
    Fellow of the Royal
    Faculty of Physicians and
    Surgeons of Glasgow

FRhL
    fetal Rhesus lung

frict
    friction

FRJM
    full range of joint
    movement

FROM
    full range of motion

FRP
    functional refractory
    period

FRS
    Fellow of the Royal Society
    furosemide

FRSC
    Fellow of the Royal Society
    (Canada)

FRSE
    Fellow of the Royal Society
    of Edinburgh

Fru
    symbol for fructose

Frust.
    L. frustillatim (in small
    pieces)

FS
    full scale (IQ)
    function study

F.s.a.
    L. fiat secundum artem (let
    it be made skillfully)

FSD
    focal skin distance

FSF
    fibrin-stabilizing factor

FSGS
    focal segmental
    glomerulosclerosis

FSH
> follicle-stimulating hormone

FSH/LH-RH
> follicle-stimulating hormone and luteinizing hormone releasing hormone

FSH-RF
> follicle-stimulating hormone releasing factor

FSH-RH
> follicle stimulating hormone releasing hormone

FSI
> foam stability index

FSMB
> Federation of State Medical Boards of the United States

FSP
> fibrin split products
> fibrinogen split products
> fibrinolytic split products

FSR
> fusiform skin revision

FSW
> field service worker

FT
> false transmitter
> family therapy
> fibrous tissue
> follow through
> Fourier transform
> full term

FT$_4$
> free thyroxine

ft.
> feet
> L. fiat or fiant (let there be made)
> foot

ft. *(continued)*
> fluorescent treponemal antibody

FTA-AB
> fluorescent treponemal antibody absorption test

FTA-ABS
> fluorescent treponemal antibody absorption test

FTBD
> full-term born dead

FTG
> full thickness graft

FTI
> free thyroxine index

FT$_3$I
> free triiodothyronine index

FTLB
> full term living birth

ft-lb
> foot-pound

FTLE
> full-thickness local excision

Ft. mas. div. in pil.
> L. fiat massa dividenda in pilulae (let a mass be made and divided into pills)

FTND
> full-term normal delivery

Ft. pulv.
> L. fiat pulvis (let a powder be made)

FTSG
> full-thickness skin graft

FTT
> failure to thrive

FU
> fecal urobilinogen
> fluorouracil

FU*(continued)*
follow-up

F/U
follow up

5-FU
fluorouracil

Fu
fluorouracil

5-Fu
fluorouracil

FUB
functional uterine bleeding

Fuc
fucose

FUDR
fluorodeoxyuridine
5-fluorouracil
deoxyribonucleoside

FUdR
fluorodeoxyuridine
5-fluorouracil
deoxyribonucleoside

FUO
fever of undetermined
origin
fever of unknown origin

FUR
fluorouracil riboside

FUTP
fluorouridine triphosphate

FUVAC
fluorouracil, vinblastine,
doxorubicin, and
cyclophosphamide

FV
facial vein
femoral vein
fluid volume

FV *(continued)*
Friend virus

fv
fever

FV-A
FV-anemia

FVC
forced vital capacity

FVC_1
1-sec forced vital capacity

FVL
femoral vein ligation

FV-P
FV-polyerythemia

F. vs.
L. fiat venaesectio (let the
patient be bled)

FW
Felix-Weil (reaction)
Folin and Wu's (method)

FWB
full weight bearing

FWHM
full width half-maximum

FWLS
fever without localizing
signs

FWR
Felix-Weil reaction

fx
fracture

Fy
blood group

FYI
for your information

FZ
focal zone

G

gauge
gauss
giga-
gingival
glucose
gonidial (colony)
good
gravida
gravitational constant
Greek
guanine
guanosine
immunoglobulin
in electrocardiography, a
symbol for ventricular
gradient, usually as
projected on the frontal
plane of the body

G

conductance
G force
Gibbs free energy
gravitational constant

G_1

symbol for the period that
follows cell division and
precedes DNA replication
in the life cycle of a cell

G_2

symbol for the period
between DNA replication
and the onset of mitosis
in the life cycle of a cell

G_{11}

hexachlorophene

g

gram
great
in electrocardiography, a
symbol for ventricular
gradient, usually as
projected on the frontal
plane of the body

g

standard gravity

Γ

gamma

γ

done
former symbol for
microgram (now µg)
the γ chains of fetal
hemoglobin
the heavy chain of IgG

GA

gastric analysis
general anesthesia
gestational age
gingivoaxial
glucuronic acid
gut-associated

Ga

gallium

GABA
γ-aminobutyric acid

GABHS
group A beta hemolytic
streptococcus

γ-Abu
γ-aminobutyric acid

GAD
glutamic acid
decarboxylase

GAF
Global Assessment of
Functioning

GAG
glycosaminoglycan

Gal
galactose

gal
    gallon

GalNAc
    N-acetylgalactosamine

gal-1-P
    galactose-1-phosphate

GALT
    gut-associated lymphoid
        tissue

GaLV
    gibbon ape lymphosarcoma
        virus

Galv.
    galvanic

GAPD
    glyceraldehyde-3-phosphate-
        dehydrogenase

GAPDH
    glyceraldehyde-3-phosphate-
        dehydrogenase

Garg.
    L. gargarismus (gargle)

GAS
    general adaptation
        syndrome

GAW
    airway conductance

Gaw
    airway conductance

GB
    gallbladder
    Guillain-Barré syndrome

GBA
    ganglionic blocking agent

GBG
    glycine-rich β glycoprotein
    properdin Factor B

GBGase
    glycine-rich β
        glycoproteinase

GBH
    graphite-benzalkonium-hep-
        arin

GBIA
    Guthrie bacterial
        inhibition assay

GBM
    glomerular basement
        membrane

GBq
    gigabecquerel

GBS
    gallbladder series
    group B streptococci

GC
    ganglion cells
    gas chromatography
    glucocorticoid
    gonoccoccus
    gonorrhea
    granular casts
    guanine cytosine

g-cal.
    gram calorie

g-cm
    gram-centimeter

GC/MS
    gas chromatography/mass
        spectroscopy

Gd
    gadolinium

GDA
    germine diacetate

GDB
    Genome Database

GDH
    glutamate dehydrogenase
    glycerophosphate
        dehydrogenase

GDM
gestational diabetes mellitus

Gdn
guanidine

GDP
guanosine diphosphate

GE
gastroenterostomy

G/E
granulocyte-erythroid ratio

Ge
germanium

Gel. quav.
L. gelatina quavis (in any kind of jelly)

geol
geological

GEP
gastroenteropancreatic

GER
gastro-esophageal reflux

GERD
gastroesophageal reflux disease

GET
gastric emptying time

GET 1/2
gastric emptying half-time

GeV
giga electron volt

Gev
giga electron volt

GF
gastric fluid
germ-free
glomerular filtration
gluten-free
grandfather

Gf
gastric fluid

GFAP
glial fibrillary acidic protein

GFCL
giant follicular cell lymphoma

GFD
gluten-free diet

GFR
glomerular filtration rate

GG
gamma globulin

GGA
general gonadotropic activity

GGE
general gland enlargement

G.G.G.
L. gummi guttae gambiae (gamboge)

GGS
glands, goiter, or stiffness

GG or S
glands, goiter, or stiffness

GGT
γ-glutamyltransferase

GGTP
gamma-glutamyl transpeptidase

GH
growth hormone

GHB
gamma hydroxy butyrate

GHD
growth hormone deficiency

GH-IH
  growth hormone inhibiting hormone

GH-RF
  growth hormone releasing factor

GH-RH
  growth hormone releasing hormone

GH-RIH
  growth hormone release inhibiting hormone

GHz
  gigahertz

GI
  gastrointestinal
  globulin insulin

GIBB
  GenInfo Backbone (database)

GIFT
  gamete intrafallopian transfer

GIGO
  garbage in, garbage out

GIK
  glucose, insulin and potassium

GIM
  gonadotropin-inhibitory material

ging
  gingiva

GIP
  gastric inhibitory polypeptide

GIS
  gas in stomach
  gastrointestinal system

GI series
  gastrointestinal series

GISSI
  Gruppo Italiano per lo Studio Della Streptochinasi Nell' Infarto Miocardico

GIT
  gastrointestinal tract

GITSG
  Gastrointestinal Tumor Study Group

GITT
  glucose-insulin tolerance test

GIX
  an insecticidal compound, DFDT

GK
  glycerol kinase

GL
  greatest length (an axis of measurement or dimension used for small flexed embryos)

Gl
  glucinium

gl
  gill

gl.
  L. glandula (gland)

g/l
  grams per liter

GL 54
  athomin

GLA
  gingivolinguoaxial

Gla
  γ-carboxyglutamic acid

GLC
  gas-liquid chromatography

Glc
  glucose

GlcA
  gluconic acid

GlcN
  glucosamine

GlcNAc
  N-acetylglucosamine

GlcUA
  glucuronic acid

GLDH
  glutamate dehydrogenase

GLI
  glucagon-like
    immunoreactivity

Gln
  glutamine
  glutaminyl

glob
  globulin

GLU
  glucose and other reducing
    agents

Glu
  glutamic acid
  glutamine

glu
  glucose

GluA
  glucuronic acid

gluc
  glucose

Glx
  symbol for glutamyl (Glu)
    and/or glutaminyl (Gln)
    to denote uncertainty
    between them

Gly
  glycine

GM
  gastric mucosa
  geometric mean
  grand mal
  grandmother
  grand multiparity
  gross motor

Gm
  gamma
  Gram stain

gm
  gram

g-m
  gram-meter

GMA
  glyceryl methacrylate

GMC
  General Medical Council
    (British)

GM-CSF
  granulocyte-macrophage
    colony-stimulationg
    factor

GMD
  glutamate dehydrogenase

GMK
  green monkey kidney
    (culture medium)

g/mL
  concentration

g/mol
  molecular weight

GMP
  guanosine monophosphate
  guanosine phosphate

3′, 5′-GMP
  cyclic guanosine
    monophosphate

GMS
  general medical services

GMS *(continued)*
Gomori's methenamine-silver (stain)

GM&S
general medicine and surgery

GMT
geometric mean titer

GMW
gram-molecular weight

GN
glomerulonephritis
glucose nitrogen (ratio)
gram negative

GNID
gram-negative intracellular diplococci

Gn-RH
gonadotropin-releasing hormone

GOE
gas, oxygen and ether

GOG
Gynecologic Oncology Group

GOK
God only knows

GOT
glutamine-oxaloacetic transaminase (aspartate aminotransferase)

govt
government

GP
general practitioner
general practitioner
glycoproteins
gram-positive
gutta percha

G6P
glucose-6-phosphate

GPAIS
guinea pig anti-insulin serum

GPC
gastric parietal cell

GPCI
geographic practice cost index

GPD
glucose phosphate dehydrogenase

G6PD
glucose-6-phosphate dehydrogenase

G6PDA
glucose-6-phosphate dehydrogenase enzyme variant A

GPDH
glucose phosphate dehydrogenase

G6PDH
glucose-6-phosphate dehydrogenase

GPI
general paralysis of the insane
glucosephosphate isomerase

GGPIMH
guinea pig intestinal mucosal homogenate

GPIPID
guinea pig intraperitoneal infectious dose

GPK
guinea pig kidney (antigen)

GPKA
guinea pig kidney absorption (test)

GPS
> guinea pig serum

GPT
> glutamic-pyruvic
> transaminase

GR
> gastric resection
> glutathione reductase

gr
> grain

GRA
> gonadotropin-releasing
> agent

Gra
> glyceraldehyde

Grad.
> L. gradatim (by degrees)

grad
> graduate

GRE
> Graduate Record
> Examination

GRF
> gonadotropin releasing
> factor
> growth hormone releasing
> factor

GRH
> growth hormone releasing
> hormone

Gri
> glyceric acid

GRID
> gay-related immune
> disease

GRIH
> growth-hormone-release-
> inhibiting hormone

Grn
> glycerone

Gro
> glycerol

GS
> general surgery

G/S
> glucose and saline

GSA
> gross virus antigen
> guanidinosuccinic acid

GSC
> gas-solid chromatography
> gravity-settling culture

GSD
> genetically significant dose
> glycogen storage disease

GSE
> gluten sensitive
> enteropathy

GSH
> reduced glutathione

GSH-Px
> glutathione peroxidase

GSR
> galvanic skin response
> generalized Shwartzman
> reaction

GSSG
> oxidized glutathione

GSSR
> generalized
> Sanarelli-Shwartzman
> reaction

GT
> generation time
> glucose tolerance
> glutamyl transpeptidase
> group therapy

gt
> great

gt.
  L. gutta (drop)

GTD
  gestational trophoblastic
    disease

GTF
  glucose tolerance factor

GTH
  gonadotropic hormone

GTN
  gestational trophoblastic
    neoplasm
  glomerulo-tubulo-nephritis
  glyceryl trinitrate

GTP
  glutamyl transpeptidase
  guanosine triphosphate

GTT
  glucose tolerance test
  oral glucose tolerance test

gtt.
  L. guttae (drops)

GU
  gastric ulcer
  genitourinary
  gonococcal urethritis

Gua
  guanine

Gul
  gulose

Guo
  guanosine

GUS
  genitourinary system

Guttat.
  L. guttatim (drop by drop)

Gutt. quibusd.
  L. guttis quibusdam (with a
    few drops)

GV
  gentian violet

GVH
  graft-versus-host (disease,
    reaction)

GVHD
  graft-versus-host disease

GVHR
  graft-versus-host reaction

GX
  glycinexylidide

GXT
  graded exercise test

Gy
  gray

gyn
  gynecologic
  gynecology

GZ
  Guilford-Zimmerman
    personality test

GZTS
  Guilford-Zimmerman
    Temperament Survey

H
  doxorubicin
    (hydroxydaunorubicin)
  hearing
  heavy
  hemagglutinin
  henry
  hernia
  heroin
  Holzknecht unit
  horizontal
  hormone
  Hounsfield unit
  hydrogen
  hypermetropia
  hyperopia
  hypodermic
  patient's home

H-1
  Parvovirus

H
  enthalpy
  Haemophilus
  Hauch (motile
    microorganism)
  magnetic field strength

H.
  L. haustus (a draft)
  L. hora (hour)

^1H
  protium (hydrogen-1)

^2H
  deuterium (hydrogen-2)

^3H
  tritium (hydrogen-3)

$[H^+]$
  hydrogen ion concentration

H_0
  null hypothesis

H_1
  alternate hypothesis

H_2
  histamine

h
  hecto-
  hour

h.
  L. hora (hour)

h
  height
  Planck's constant

HA
  hallux abductus
  headache
  height age
  hemadsorbent
  hemagglutinating antibody
  hemagglutination
  hemagglutinin
  hemolytic anemia
  hepatic artery
  hospital admission
  hydroxyapatite

Ha
  hahnium

HAA
  hepatitis-associated
    antigen

HABA
  hydroxybenzeneazobenzoic
    acid

habit
  habitat

HAc
  acetic acid

HACS
  hyperactive child
    syndrome

HAD
  hemadsorption

HAD *(continued)*
  hexamethylmelamine, doxorubicin, and cisplatin

HAE
  hereditary angioedema

HAFOE
  high air flow oxygen enrichment

HAGG
  hyperimmune antivariola gamma globulin

HAHTG
  horse antihuman thymus globulin

HAI
  hemagglutination inhibition
  hemagglutinin inhibition
  hepatic artery infusion

hal
  halothane

HAM
  human albumin microspheres

HANE
  hereditary angioneurotic edema

HANES
  Health and Nutrition Examination Survey

HAP
  haptoglobin
  heredopathia atactica polyneuritiformis
  histamine phosphate acid
  hydroxyapatite

HAPA
  hemagglutinating antipenicillin antibody

HAPC
  hospital-acquired penetration contact

HAPE
  high-altitude pulmonary edema

Har
  homoarginine

HASHD
  hypertensive arteriosclerotic heart disease

HAT
  hypoxanthine-aminopterin-thymidine (medium)

Haust.
  L. haustus (a draft)

HAV
  hepatitis A virus

HB
  heart block
  hepatitis B
  highball
  housebound

HB_c
  hepatitis B core (antigen)

HB_e
  hepatitis B e (antigen)

HB_s
  hepatitis B surface (antigen)

Hb
  hemoglobin

H-2b
  mouse cells

HB_cAb
  antibody to the hepatitis B core antigen

HB_eAb
  antibody to the hepatitis B e antigen

HB$_s$Ab
  antibody to the hepatitis B
  surface antigen

HBABA
  hydroxybenzeneazobenzoic
  acid

HB-Ag
  hepatitis B antigen

HB$_c$Ag
  hepatitis B core antigen

HB$_e$Ag
  hepatitis B e antigen

HB$_s$Ag
  hepatitis B surface
  (antigen)

HbAS
  heterozygosity for
  hemoglobin A and
  hemoglobin S, the sickle
  cell trait

HBB
  hydroxybenzyl
  benzimidazole

Hb Barts
  Bart's hemoglobin

HbCO
  carboxyhemoglobin

HbCV
  Haemophilus influenzae b
  conjugate vaccine
  hepatitis B conjugate
  vaccine

HBD
  hydroxybutyric
  dehydrogenase

HBDH
  α-hydroxybutyrate
  dehydrogenase

HBF
  hepatic blood flow

Hb F
  fetal hemoglobin

HBI
  high serum-bound iron

HBIG
  hepatitis B immune
  globulin

HBLV
  human B lymphotropic
  virus

HBO
  hyperbaric oxygenation

HbO$_2$
  oxyhemoglobin

HbOC
  oligosaccharide-CRM$_{197}$
  conjugate *Haemophilus
  influenzae* b vaccine

HBP
  high blood pressure

HbPV
  Haemophilus influenzae b
  polysaccharide vaccine

HBr
  hydrobromic acid

Hb S
  sickle cell hemoglobin

HBSS
  Hank's balanced salt
  solution

HBV
  hepatitis B virus

HBW
  high birth weight

HC
  hair cell
  handicapped
  head circumference
  head compression
  heparin cofactor

HC *(continued)*
    hepatic catalase
    hospital corps
    house call
    Huntington's chorea
    hyaline casts
    hydrocortisone
    hydroxycorticoid

Hc
    hematocrit

H-CAP
    hexamethylmelamine,
    cyclophosphamide,
    doxorubicin, and cisplatin

HCC
    hepatocellular carcinoma
    hydroxycholecalciferol

HCD
    heavy chain disease

HCFA
    Health Care Financing
    Administration

HCG
    human chorionic
    gonadotropin

hCG
    human chorionic
    gonadotropin

HCH
    hexachlorocyclohexane

HCHO
    formaldehyde

HCL
    hairy cell leukemia

HCl
    hydrochloric acid
    hydrochloride

HCMV
    human cytomegalovirus

HCN
    hydrocyanic acid

HCN *(continued)*
    hydrogen cyanide

HCO_3
    the bicarbonate radical

HCP
    hepatocatalase peroxidase
    hereditary coproporphyria

HCS
    human chorionic
      somatomammotropic
      hormone
    human chorionic
      somatomammotropin

17-HCS
    17-hydroxycorticosteroids

hCS
    human chorionic
      somatomammotropin

HCT
    hematocrit
    homocytotrophic
    human chorionic
      thyrotropin
    hydrochlorothiazide

Hct
    hematocrit

hCT
    human calcitonin

HCTU
    home cervical traction unit

HCTZ
    hydrochlorothiazide

HCU
    homocystinuria

HCV
    hepatitis C virus
    human coronavirus

HCVD
    hypertensive
      cardiovascular disease

HCW
    health care worker

Hcy
    homocysteine

HD
    head
    hearing distance
    heart disease
    hemodialysis
    high dosage
    hip disarticulation
    Hodgkin's disease
    hydatid disease

H.D.
    L. heloma durum (hard
        corn)

H.d.
    L. hora decubitus (at
        bedtime)

HDC
    histidine decarboxylase

HDCV
    human diploid cell rabies
        vaccine

HDF
    high dry field

HDH
    heart disease history

HDL
    high-density lipoprotein

HDL$_1$
    Lp(a) lipoprotein

HDL-C
    HDL-cholesterol

HDLP
    high-density lipoprotein

HDLW
    hearing distance for watch
        in left ear

HDN
    hemolytic disease of the
        newborn

HDP
    hydroxydimethylpyrim-
        idine

HDR
    Harrington distraction rod

HDRV
    human diploid cell rabies
        vaccine

HDRW
    hearing distance for watch
        in right ear

HDS
    herniated disk syndrome

HDU
    hemodialysis unit

HDV
    hepatitis D virus
    human delta virus

HE
    hereditary elliptocytosis
    human enteric

H and E
    hematoxylin and eosin
        (stain)

H&E
    hematoxylin and eosin
        (stain)

He
    helium

^{3}He
    helium-3

^{4}He
    helium-4

HEAT
    human erythrocyte
        agglutination test

Hebdom.
    L. hebdomada (a week)

HEC
hydroxyergocalciferol

HED
unit of roentgen-ray dosage
(Ger. Haut-Einheits
Dosis)

HEDTA
N-hydroxyethylethylenedi-
aminetriacetic acid

HEENT
head, eyes, ears, nose and
throat

HEK
human embryo kidney (cell
culture)
human embryonic kidney

HEL
human embryo lung (cell
culture)

HeLa cells
cells of the first
continuously cultured
(human cervical)
carcinoma strain

HEMPAS
hereditary erythroblastic
multinuclearity
associated with positive
acidified serum

HEPA
high-efficiency particulate
air (filter)

HEPT
1-(2-hydroxyethoxymethyl)-
6-phenylthiothymine

Herb. recent.
L. herbarium recentium (of
fresh herbs)

HES
hydroxyethyl starch

HET
helium equilibration time

HETE
hydroxyeicosatetraenoic
acid

HETP
hexaethyltetraphosphate

HEV
hemagglutinating
encephalomyelitis virus
high endothelial venules

HEW
Department of Health
Education and Welfare
(now Department of
Health and Human
Services, HHS)

HexaCAF
hexamethylmelamine,
cyclophosphamide,
doxorubicin, and
5-fluorouracil

HF
Hageman factor
(coagulation Factor XII)
hay fever
heart failure
hemorrhagic fever
high flow
high frequency

Hf
hafnium

HFFTTA
hypermobile flat foot with
tight tendo Achillis

HFI
hereditary fructose
intolerance

H$_4$folate
tetrahydrofolate

HFP
hexafluoropropylene

Hfr
   high-frequency
      recombination

Hg
   hemoglobin
   mercury (L. hydrargyrum)

hg
   hectogram
   hyperglycemic factor

Hgb
   hemoglobin

HGA
   homogentisic acid

HGF
   hyperglycemic-glycogeno-
      lytic factor (glucagon)

HGG
   human gamma globulin

HGH
   human (pituitary) growth
      hormone

hGH
   human (pituitary) growth
      hormone

hGHr
   growth hormone
      recombinant

Hg(NO$_3$)$_2$
   mercuric nitrate

HGP
   Human Genome Project

HGPRT
   hypoxanthine-guanine
      phosphoribosyltransferase

HGPRTase
   hypoxanthine-guanine
      phosphoribosyltrans-
      ferase

HH
   hiatus hernia
   hydroxyhexamide

H&H
   hemoglobin and
      hematocrit

H-H
   Henderson-Hasselbalch
      (equation)

HHA
   hereditary hemolytic
      anemia
   home health agency

HHb
   deoxyhemoglobin
   un-ionized hemoglobin

HHD
   hypertensive heart disease

H and Hm
   compound hypermetropic
      astigmatism

HHNK
   hyperglycemic,
      hyperosmolar, nonketotic
      (coma)

HHS
   Department of Health and
      Human Services
   Harris hip score

HHT
   hereditary hemorrhagic
      telangiectasis
   hydroxyheptadecatrienoic
      acid

HHV6
   human herpesvirus 6

HI
   hemagglutination
      inhibition

HIA
   hemagglutination
      inhibition antibody

5-HIAA
   5-hydroxyindoleacetic acid

HIB
  Haemophilus influenzae
  type B

H-ICDA
  hospital adaptation of
  ICDA

HID
  headache, insomnia,
  depression

HIG
  hemolysis in gel

HIHA
  high impulsiveness, high
  anxiety

HILA
  high impulsiveness, low
  anxiety

HIMA
  Health Industry
  Manufacturers
  Association

HIOMT
  hydroxyindole-*o*-methyl
  transferase

Hip
  hip amputation

HIS
  hospital information
  system

His
  histidine

HIT
  hemagglutination-inhibition
  test
  home intravenous therapy
  hypertrophic infiltrative
  tendinitis

HIV
  human immunodeficiency
  virus

HIVAT
  home intravenous
  antibiotic therapy

HIVIG
  hyperimmune intravenous
  (immuno)globulin

HJ
  hepatojugular
  Howell-Jolly (bodies)

HJB
  Howell-Jolly bodies

HJR
  hepatojugular reflex

HK
  heat-killed
  hexokinase

HKAFO
  hip-knee-ankle-foot
  orthosis

HKLM
  heat-killed *Listeria
  monocytogenes*

HL
  half life
  hearing level
  hearing loss
  histiocytic lymphoma
  histocompatibility locus
  hypermetropia, latent

H&L
  heart and lungs

Hl
  latent hyperopia

hl
  hectoliter

HLA
  human leukocyte antigen
  human lymphocyte antigen

HLDH
  heat-stable lactic
  dehydrogenase

hLH
  human luteinizing
    hormone

HLK
  heart, liver, kidney

HLP
  hyperlipoproteinemia

hLT
  human lymphocyte
    transformation

HLV
  herpes-like virus

HM
  hand movement
  heart murmur
  L. heloma molle (soft corn)
  human milk
  hydatidiform mole

Hm
  manifest hyperopia

hm
  hectometer

HMB
  homatropine methyl
    bromide

HMD
  hyaline membrane disease

HMF
  hydroxymethylfurfural

HMG
  human menopausal
    gonadotropin
  hydroxymethylglutaryl

hMG
  human menopausal
    gonadotropin

HMG-CoA
  3-hydroxy-3-methylglutaryl-
    coenzyme A

HML
  human milk lysozyme

HMM
  hexamethylmelamine

Hmm
  hexamethylmelamine

HMO
  health maintenance
    organization

HMP
  hexose monophosphate
  hexose monophosphate
    pathway
  hot moist packs

HMPG
  4-hydroxy-3-methoxy-
    phenyl ethylene glycol

HMPS
  hexose monophosphate
    shunt

HMR
  histiocytic medullary
    reticulosis

HMS
  hypothetical mean strain

HMSA
  (Medicare) Health
    Manpower Shortage Area

HMSAS
  hypertrophic muscular
    subaortic stenosis

HMW
  high molecular weight

HMW-NCF
  high-molecular-weight
    neutrophil chemotactic
    factor

HMX
  heat-massage-exercise

HN
  hereditary nephritis
  hilar node

HN2
nitrogen mustard

HN₂
nitrogen mustard, mechlorethamine

HNP
herniated nucleus pulposus

hnRNA
heterogeneous nuclear RNA

HNSHA
hereditary nonsperocytic hemolytic anemia

HNV
has not voided

HO
house officer
high oxygen
hyperbaric oxygen

H₂O
water

H₂O₂
hydrogen peroxide

H/O
history of

Ho
holmium

HOB
head of bed

HOC
hydroxycorticoid

HOCM
hypertrophic obstructive cardiomyopathy

HOH
hard of hearing

HOOD
hereditary osteo-onychodysplasia

HOP
high oxygen pressure
hydroxydaunomycin (doxorubicin), Oncovin (vincristine), and prednisone

Hor. decub.
L. hora decubitus (at bedtime)

Hor. interm.
L. horis intermediis (at the intermediate hours)

Hor. som.
at bedtime (hora somni)

Hor. un. spatio
L. horae unius spatio (at the end of one hour)

hosp
hospitalization

HOT
human old tuberculin

HP
high protein
hot packs
house physician
human pituitary

H + P
(medical) history and physical (examination)

H&P
history and physical

Hp
haptoglobin

HPA
hypothalamic-pituitary-adrenal

HPAA
hydroxyphenylacetic acid

Hpb
haptoglobin

HPE
history and physical examination

HPETE
hydroperoxyeicosatetra-enoic acid

HPF
heparin-precipitable fraction
high-power field

HPFH
hereditary persistence of fetal hemoglobin

hPFSH
human pituitary follicle-stimulating hormone

HPG
human pituitary gonadotropin

hPG
human pituitary gonadotropin

HPI
history of present illness

HPL
human placental lactogen

hPL
human placental lactogen

HPLA
hydroxyphenyllactic acid

HPLC
high-pressure liquid chromatography
high-performance liquid chromatography

HPO
high-pressure oxygenation

HPP
hydroxypyrazolopymidine

HPPA
hydroxyphenylpyruvic acid

HPPH
hydroxyphenylphenylhydan-toin

HPRT
hypoxanthine phosphoribosyltrans-ferase

HPS
hematoxylin-phyloxine-saffron
hypertrophic pyloric stenosis

HPT
hyperparathyroidism

HPV
Haemophilus pertussis vaccine
human papillomavirus

HPVD
hypertensive pulmonary vascular disease

HPVG
hepatic portal venous gas

Hpx
hemopexin

H₂Q
ubiquinol

HR
heart rate
hormone receptor
hospital record

H&R
hysterectomy and radiation

Hr
blood type factor

hr
hour

HRA
    Health Resources
        Administration
    health risk appraisal

HRBC
    horse red blood cells

HRF
    histamine releasing factor

HRIG
    human rabies immune
        globulin

HRL
    head rotated left

HRR
    head rotated right

HRS
    Hamilton Rating Scale

HRSA
    Health Resources and
        Services Administration

HRT
    heart rate

HS
    half strength
    heart sounds
    heat-stable
    heme synthetase
    hereditary spherocytosis
    herpes simplex
    high school
    homosexual
    horse serum
    house surgeon
    Hurler's syndrome

h.s.
    L. hora somni (at bedtime)

H&S
    hysterectomy and
        sterilization

HSA
    human serum albumin
    hypersomnia-sleep apnea

HSC
    Hand-Schüller-Christian
        disease

HSCA
    Health Sciences
        Communications
        Association

HSE
    herpes simplex
        encephalitis

Hse
    homoserine

HSF
    hydrazine-sensitive factor

HSG
    herpes simplex genitalis
    hysterosalpingogram

HSL
    herpes simplex labialis

HSQB
    Health Standards Quality
        Bureau

HSR
    homogeneously staining
        regions

HSRA
    Health Services and
        Resources Administration

HSV
    herpes simplex virus

HSV I
    herpes simplex virus type I

HSV II
    herpes simplex virus type
        II

HT
    hammertoe
    heart
    height
    hemagglutination titer

HT *(continued)*
    histologic technician
    Hubbard tank
    hypermetropia, total
    hypertension
    hypodermic tablet

5-HT
    5-hydroxytryptamine
      (serotonin)

Ht
    heart
    heat
    height
    hot
    total hyperopia

HTA
    hydroxytryptamine

HTACS
    human thyroid adenylate
      cyclase stimulators

HTC
    homozygous typing cells

H-TGL
    hepatic triglyceride lipase

HTHD
    hypertensive heart disease

HTLV
    human T-cell
      leukemia/lymphoma
      virus

HTLV-III
    human T-cell lymphotropic
      virus type III

HTN
    hypertension

htn
    hypertension

HTP
    hydroxytryptophan

HTR
    hemolytic transfusion
      reaction

HTV
    herpes-type virus

HU
    heat unit
    hemagglutinating unit
    hydroxyurea
    hyperemia unit

HuIFN
    human interferon

HUS
    hemolytic-uremic
      syndrome
    hyaluronidase unit for
      semen

HUTHAS
    human thymus antiserum

HV
    hallux valgus
    hepatic vein
    herpesvirus
    hyperventilation

H and V
    hemigastrectomy and
      vagotomy

HVA
    homovanillic acid

HVD
    hypertensive vascular
      disease

HVE
    high-voltage
      electrophoresis

HVH
    herpesvirus hominis

HVL
    half-value layer

HVSD
    hydrogen-detected
      ventricular septal defect

Hx
    hexyl

Hx *(continued)*
    history
    hemopexin

Hy
    hypermetropia

Hyl
    hydroxylysine
    hydroxylysyl

Hyp
    hydroxyproline
    hypoxanthine

hyp
    hypodermic

Hyst
    hysterectomy

Hyster
    hysterectomy

HZ
    herpes zoster

Hz
    hertz

HZV
    herpes zoster virus

I
incisor
inosine
intensity of magnetism
intercalary (congenital
absence of limb)
iodine

I
electric current
intensity (of radiant
energy)
ionic strength

^{125}I
iodine-125

^{131}I
iodine-131

i
deciduous incisor
optically inactive

IA
impedance angle
internal auditory
intra-aortic
intra-arterial

Ia
I-region antigen

IABP
intra-aortic balloon pump

IAC
internal auditory canal

IACR
International Association
of Cancer Registries

IADH
inappropriate antidiuretic
hormone

IADHS
inappropriate antidiuretic
hormone syndrome

IADR
International Association
for Dental Research

IAEA
International Atomic
Energy Agency

IAET
International Association
for Enterostomal Therapy

IAGP
International Association
of Geographic Pathology

IAH
idiopathic adrenal
hyperplasia

IAHA
immune adherence
hemagglutination assay

IAM
internal auditory meatus

IANC
International Anatomical
Nomenclature Committee

IAO
immediately after onset

IAP
intermittent acute
porphyria
International Academy of
Pathology

IARC
International Agency for
Research on Cancer

IAS
interatrial septum
intra-amniotic saline
infusion

IASD
   interatrial septal defect

IAT
   intraoperative autologous
      transfusion
   invasive activity test
   iodine-azide test

IB
   immune body
   inclusion body

IBB
   intestinal brush border

IBC
   iron-binding capacity

IBF
   immunoglobulin-binding
      factor

IBI
   intermittent bladder
      irrigation

ibid
   ibidem (at the same place)

IBM
   inclusion body myositis

IBR
   infectious bovine
      rhinotracheitis

IBS
   irritable bowel syndrome

IBSN
   infantile bilateral striatal
      necrosis

IBU
   international benzoate unit

IBV
   infectious bronchitis virus

IBW
   ideal body weight

IC
   immune complexes

IC *(continued)*
   inspiratory capacity
   integrated circuit
   intensive care
   intercostal
   intermediate care
   intermittent claudication
   internal capsule
   internal conversion
   intracarotid
   intracavitary
   intracellular
   intracoronary
   intracranial
   intracutaneous
   irritable colon
   isovolumic contraction

i.c.
   intracerebral

ICA
   ileocolic anastomosis
   internal carotid artery
   intracranial aneurysm

ICAO
   internal carotid artery
      occlusion

ICB
   intercostal nerve block

ICC
   immunocompetent cells
   Indian childhood cirrhosis
   intensive coronary care
   Interstate Commerce
      Commission

ICCU
   intensive coronary care
      unit

ICD
   International Classification
      of Diseases
   intrauterine contraceptive
      device
   ischemic coronary disease
   isocitrate dehydrogenase
   isocitric dehydrogenase

ICDA

International Classification
of Diseases and Accidents
International Classification
of Diseases, Adapted for
Use in the United States

ICF

intermediate care facility
intracellular fluid

ICFA

incomplete Freund's
adjuvant

ICG

indocyanine green

ICM

intercostal margin

ICN

International Council of
Nurses

ICNND

Interdepartmental
Committee on Nutrition
in National Defense

ICP

intracranial pressure

ICRP

International Commission
on Radiological
Protection

ICRU

International Commission
on Radiological Units and
Measurements

ICS

Beckman
Immunochemistry
System
intercostal space
International College of
Surgeons

ICSH

International Committee
for Standardization in
Hematology
interstitial
cell–stimulating hormone
(luteinizing hormone)

ICSP

International Council of
Societies of Pathology

ICT

indirect Coombs' test
inflammation of connective
tissue
insulin coma therapy
intermittent cervical
traction
isovolumic contraction
time

ICU

intensive care unit

ICW

intracellular water

IC wave

isovolumetric contraction
wave

ID

identification
immunodiffusion
infectious disease
infective dose
inside diameter
intradermal
intraduodenal

ID$_{50}$

median infective dose

I&D

incision and drainage

Id

India
Indian

Id.
> L. idem (the same)

IDA
> image display and analysis
> iron deficiency anemia

IDD
> insulin-dependent diabetes

IDDM
> insulin-dependent diabetes
> mellitus

IDE
> investigational device
> exemption

idem
> the same (author)

IDI
> induction-delivery interval

IDK
> internal derangement of
> the knee

IDL
> intermediate-density
> lipoprotein

IDM
> infant of a diabetic mother

IDMS
> isotope dilution-mass
> spectrometry

Ido
> idose

IDP
> inosine 5′-diphosphate

IDR
> intradermal reaction

IDS
> immunity deficiency state
> inhibitor of DNA synthesis

IDU
> idoxuridine
> iododeoxyuridine

IDV
> intermittent demand
> ventilation

IDVC
> indwelling venous catheter

IE
> immunizing unit (Ger.
> immunitäts Einheit)
> immunoelectrophoresis

i.e.
> L. id est (that is)

IEF
> isoelectric focusing

IEM
> immune electron
> microscopy
> inborn error of metabolism

IEMG
> integrated electromyogram

IEP
> immunoelectrophoresis
> isoelectric point
> isoelectric precipitation

I/E ratio
> inspiratory to expiratory
> ratio

I:E ratio
> inspiratory to expiratory
> ratio

IF
> immunofixation
> immunofluorescence
> interferon
> interstitial fluid
> intrinsic factor
> involved field (irradiation)

IFA
> indirect fluorescent
> antibody test

IFC
> intrinsic factor concentrate

IFCC
International Federation of Clinical Chemistry

IFE
immunofixation electrophoresis

IFN
interferon

IFR
inspiratory flow rate

IFRA
indirect fluorescent rabies antibody (test)

IFV
intracellular fluid volume

IG
immune globulin
intragastric

Ig
immunoglobulin

IgA
immunoglobulin A

IgD
immunoglobulin D

IGDM
infant of gestational diabetic mother

IgE
immunoglobulin E

IGF
insulin-like growth factor

IgG
immunoglobulin G

IgM
immunoglobulin M

IGT
impaired glucose tolerance

IGTN
ingrown toenail

IGV
intrathoracic gas volume

IH
infectious hepatitis
inpatient hospital

IHA
indirect hemagglutination

IHBTD
incompatible hemolytic blood transfusion disease

IHC
idiopathic hypercalciuria

IHD
ischemic heart disease

IHO
idiopathic hypertrophic osteoarthropathy

IHR
intrinsic heart rate

IHS
Indian Health Service

IHSA
radioactive iodine-tagged human serum albumin

IHSS
idiopathic hypertrophic subaortic stenosis

IHW
inner heel wedge

IIF
indirect immunofluorescent

IJP
internal jugular pressure

IJV
internal jugular vein

IL
independent laboratory
interleukin

Il
illinium

ILA
insulin-like activity
International Leprosy
Association

ILD
ischemic leg disease
ischemic limb disease

Ile
isoleucine

IM
infectious mononucleosis
intermuscular
internal medicine
intramedullary
intramuscular
intramuscularly (by
intramuscular injection)

IMA
internal mammary artery

IMAA
iodinated macroaggregated
albumin

IMB
intermenstrual bleeding

IMBC
indirect maximum
breathing capacity

ImD$_{50}$
median immunizing dose

IMF
intermaxillary fixation

IMH
idiopathic myocardial
hypertrophy

IMHP
1-iodomercuri-2-hydroxy-
propane

IMI
inferior mycoardial
infarct(ion)
intramuscular injection
intramuscular injection

IMMC
interdigestive migratory
motor complex

IMP
impression
improved
inosine monophosphate

IMPA
incisal mandibular plane
angle

IMR
infant mortality rate

IMS
incurred in military
service

IMV
intermittent mandatory
ventilation

IMViC
indole, methyl red,
Voges-Proskauer, citrate

imvic
indole, methyl red,
Voges-Proskauer, citrate

IN
intranasal

In
inch
indium

in.
inch

i.n.
intranasal

INA
>International Neurological
>Association

INAD
>infantile neuroaxonal
>dystrophy

INAH
>isoniazid acid hydrazide
>isonicotinic acid hydrazide

INC
>increase

inc
>increase

INCAP
>Institute of Nutrition of
>Central America and
>Panama

incl
>including

incompat
>incompatibility

INCR
>increase

IND
>Investigational New Drug
>(Application)

in d.
>L. in dies (daily)

INDM
>infant of nondiabetic
>mother

indust
>industrial
>industry

INE
>infantile necrotizing
>encephalomyelopathy

Inf
>infant
>infected

Inf *(continued)*
>inferior
>infusion

Inf.
>L. infunde (pour in)

INFH
>ischemic necrosis of
>femoral head

info
>information

ING
>inguinal

ing
>inguinal

INH
>trademark for isonicotine
>hydrazine (isoniazid)

inhib
>inhibition
>inhibitor

inj
>inject
>injected
>injury

Inj. enem.
>L. injiciatur enema (let an
>enema be injected)

INN
>International
>Nonproprietary Name

INO
>internuclear
>ophthalmoplegia

Ino
>inosine

inorg
>inorganic

INPV
>intermittent
>negative-pressure
>assisted ventilation

INS
idiopathic nephrotic
syndrome

insol
insoluble

InsP$_3$
inositol 1,4,5-triphosphate

INSS
International Staging
System (for
neuroblastoma)

inst
institute

int
internal

int. cib.
L. inter cibos (between
meals)

intern
internal

intest
intestinal
intestine

Intl
International

intox
intoxication

IO
inferior oblique
internal os
intestinal obstruction
intraocular

I&O
input and output

I/O
input/output

Io
ionium

IOFB
intraocular foreign body

IOI
intraosseous infusion

IOL
intraocular lens

IOP
intraocular pressure

IP
incisoproximal
incubation period
inosine phosphorylase
instantaneous pressure
interphalangeal
intraperitoneally
isoelectric point

IP$_3$
inositol 1,4,5-triphosphate

IPAA
International
Psychoanalytical
Association

I-para
primipara

IPC
intraperitoneal
chemotherapy
isopropyl chlorophenyl

IPD
inflammatory pelvic
disease
intermittent peritoneal
dialysis

IPG
impedance
plethysmograph
impedance
plethysmography
gradient

IPH
idiopathic pulmonary
hemosiderosis

IPJ
interphalangeal joint

IPK
    intractable plantar
    keratosis

IPL
    intrapleural

IPN
    infectious pancreatic
    necrosis
    Intern's progress note

IPP
    intermittent positive
    pressure

IPPB
    intermittent positive
    pressure breathing

IPPI
    interruption of pregnancy
    for psychiatric indication

IPPO
    intermittent positive
    pressure inflation with
    oxygen

IPPR
    intermittent positive
    pressure respiration

IPPV
    intermittent positive
    pressure ventilation

iPrSGal
    isopropylthiogalactoside

IPS
    inferior petrosal sinus
    initial prognostic score

Ips
    pipsyl (p-iodophenyl
    sulfonyl)

IPSID
    immunoproliferative small
    intestinal disease

IPSP
    inhibitory postsynaptic
    potential

IPTG
    isopropylthiogalactoside

IPV
    poliovirus vaccine
    inactivated

IQ
    intelligence quotient

IR
    immune response
    immunoreactive
    index of response
    inferior rectus
    infrared
    internal resistance

Ir
    iridium

IRA
    ileorectal anastomosis

IRBBB
    incomplete right bundle
    branch block

IRC
    inspiratory reserve
    capacity

IRDS
    idiopathic respiratory
    distress syndrome
    infant respiratory distress
    syndrome

IRE
    internal rotation in
    extension

IRF
    internal rotation in flexion

IRG
    immunoreactive glucagon

Ir genes
    immune response genes

IRHCS
immunoradioassayable human chorionic somatomammotropin

IRhGH
immunoreactive human growth hormone

IRI
immunoreactive insulin

IRIS
International Research Information Service

IRMA
immunoradiometric assay
intraretinal microvascular abnormalities

IRR
intra-renal reflux

irr
irradiation

IRS
infrared spectrophotometry

IRV
inspiratory reserve volume

IR wave
isovolumetric relaxation wave

IS
immune serum
intercostal space
interspace
intraspinal

ISA
intrinsic sympathomimetic activity

ISC
irreversible sickle cell

ISCLT
International Society for Clinical Laboratory Technology

ISCP
International Society of Comparative Pathology

ISCV
International Society for Cardiovascular Surgery

ISD
isosorbide dinitrate

ISDN
isosorbide dinitrate

ISE
ion-selective electrode

ISF
interstitial fluid

ISG
immune serum globulin

ISGE
International Society of Gastroenterology

ISH
icteric serum hepatitis
International Society of Hematology

ISM
International Society of Microbiologists

ISN
intussusception

ISO
International Standards Organization

iso
isoproterenol

isoln
isolation

ISP
   interspace

IST
   insulin sensitivity test
   insulin shock therapy

ISU
   International Society of
      Urology

ISW
   interstitial water

IT
   implantation test
   inhalation test
   inhalation therapy
   intensive therapy
   intradermal test
   intrathecal
   intratracheal
   intratracheal tube
   intratumoral
   isomeric transition

ITA
   International Tuberculosis
      Association

ITC
   imidazolyl-thioguanine
      chemotherapy

IαTI
   inter-α-trypsin inhibitor

ITLC
   instant thin-layer
      chromatography

ITP
   idiopathic
      thrombocytopenic
      purpura
   immune thrombocytopenic
      purpura
   inosine triphosphate

ITT
   insulin tolerance test
   internal tibial torsion

IU
   immunizing unit
   international unit
   intrauterine

IUB
   International Union of
      Biochemistry

IUC
   International Union of
      Chemistry

IUCD
   intrauterine contraceptive
      device

IUD
   intrauterine
      (contraceptive) device
   intrauterine death

IUDR
   idoxuridine
      (5-iododeoxyuridine)

IUGR
   intrauterine growth rate
   intrauterine growth
      retardation

IUM
   intrauterine fetally
      malnourished

IUPAC
   International Union of
      Pure and Applied
      Chemistry

IUT
   intrauterine transfusion

IV
   interventricular
   intervertebral
   intravascular
   intravenous
   intravenously (by
      intravenous injection)
   intravertebral
   invasive

I-V
intraventricular

IVag
intravaginal

IVAP
in vivo adhesive platelet

IVC
inferior vena cava
intravenous cholangiogram

IVCC
intravascular consumption
coagulopathy

IVCD
intraventricular
conduction defect
intraventricular
conduction delay

IVCP
inferior vena cava pressure

IVCV
inferior venacavography

IVD
intervertebral disk

IVDU
intravenous drug user

IVF
intravascular fluid
in-vitro fertilization

IVGTT
intravenous glucose
tolerance test

IVH
intraventricular
hemorrhage

IVIG
intravenous
immunoglobulin

IVJC
intervertebral joint
complex

IVM
intravascular mass

IVP
intravenous push
intravenous pyelogram
intravenous pyelography
intraventricular pressure

IVPB
intravenous piggyback

IVPF
isovolume pressure flow
curve

IVS
interventricular septum

IVSD
interventricular septal
defect

IVT
intravenous transfusion

IVTTT
intravenous tolbutamide
tolerance test

IVU
intravenous urography

IWL
insensible water loss

IWMI
inferior wall myocardial
infarction

J
 Jewish
 joint
 joule
 Journal
 juice

J
 flux

JAMA
 Journal of the American
 Medical Association

JBE
 Japanese B encephalitis

JBJS
 Journal of Bone and Joint
 Surgery

JCAH
 Joint Commission on
 Accreditation of Hospitals

JCAHO
 Joint Commission on the
 Accreditation of
 Healthcare Organizations

JCAHPO
 Joint Commission on
 Allied Health Personnel
 in Ophthalmology

JCI
 Journal of Clinical
 Investigation

JCV
 JC virus

JEJ
 jejunum

JEM
 Journal of Experimental
 Medicine

JFS
 Jewish Family Service

JG
 juxtaglomerular

JGC
 juxtaglomerular cell

JGI
 juxtaglomerular
 granulation index

JJ
 jaw jerk

Jk
 Kidd blood group

JNA
 Jena Nomina Anatomica,
 1935

JND
 just noticeable difference

jnt
 joint

JODM
 juvenile onset diabetes
 mellitus

JPC
 junctional premature
 contraction

JPET
 Journal of Pharmacology
 and Experimental
 Therapeutics

JPS
 joint position sense

JRA
 juvenile rheumatoid
 arthritis

JT
 joint
 junctional tachycardia

Jts
> joints

juscul.
> L. jusculum (soup or broth)

juv
> juvenile

JV
> jugular vein
> jugular venous

JVD
> jugular venous distension

JVP
> jugular venous pulse

K
    absolute zero
    calix
    electrostatic capacity
    Kell blood system
    kelvin
    kidney
    phylloquinone
    potassium (L. kalium)
    thousand
    time

K
    empirical factor
    equilibrium constant

K_a
    acid dissociation constant

K_b
    base dissociation constant

K_d
    dissociation constant

K_{eq}
    equilibrium constant

K_M
    Michaelis constant

K_m
    Michaelis constant

K_{sp}
    solubility product constant

K_W
    the ion product of water

k
    kilo-

k
    Boltzmann's constant
    glass electrode constant
    rate constant
    K and k blood groups

κ
    one of the two types of
        immunoglobulin light
        chains

KA
    ketoacidosis
    King-Armstrong (units)

KAF
    conglutinogen activating
        factor (factor I)

KAFO
    knee-ankle-foot orthosis

kat
    katal

KAU
    King-Armstrong units

KB
    ketone bodies

Kb
    kilobase (1000 base pairs)

kbp
    kilo base pair(s)

KBr
    potassium bromide

KC
    cathodal (kathodal) closing
    Kupffer cells

kc
    kilocycle

kcal
    kilocalorie

KCC
    cathodal (kathodal)-closing
        contraction

K cell
    killer cell

157

KCG
    kinetocardiogram

kCi
    kilocurie

KCl
    potassium chloride

kcps
    kilocycles per second

KCS
    keratoconjunctivitis sicca

KCT
    cathodal (kathodal) closure
        tetanus

KD
    cathodal (kathodal)
        duration

KDC
    independent kidney disease
        treatment center

KDT
    kathodal (cathodal)
        duration tetanus

Ke
    an antigenic marker
        distinguishing human
        immunoglobulin λ light
        chain subtypes

K-el
    phyllochromenol

keV
    kilo electron volt

kev
    kilo electron volt

KFAB
    kidney-fixing antibody

KFD
    Kyasanur Forest disease

KFS
    Klippel-Feil syndrome

kg
    kilogram

αKG
    α-ketoglutarate

kg-cal
    kilogram-calorie

KGS
    ketogenic steroid

KHN
    Knoop hardness number

kHz
    kilohertz

KI
    karyopyknotic index
    potassium iodide

KIA
    Kliger iron agar

KIU
    kallikrein-inhibiting unit

KJ
    kilojoule

kj
    knee jerk

KK
    knee kick

kk
    knee kick

kl
    kiloliter

Kleb
    Klebsiella

KLH
    keyhole-limpet
        hemocyanin

KLS
    kidney, liver, spleen

KM
    kanamycin

Km
    Michaelis constant

km
    kilometer

KMnO
    potassium permanganate

KMV
    killed measles virus
        vaccine

KN
    knee

Kn
    know
    knowledge

KO
    knocked out (rendered
        unconscious)

KOC
    cathodal (kathodal)
        opening contraction

KOH
    potassium hydroxide

KP
    keratitic precipitates
    keratitis punctata

KPA
    prourokinase (kidney
        plasminogen activator)

kPa
    kilopascal

KPTT
    kaolin partial
        thromboplastin time

kQW-hr
    kilowatt-hour

Kr
    krypton

KRB
    Krebs-Ringer bicarbonate
        buffer

KRP
    Kolmer's test with Reiter
        protein
    Krebs-Ringer phosphate

KS
    ketosteroid
    Klinefelter's syndrome
    Kveim-Siltzbach (test)

KSC
    cathodal (kathodal) closing
        contraction

KSS
    Kearns-Sayre syndrome

KST
    cathodal (kathodal) closing
        tetanus

KU
    Karmen units

KUB
    kidney, ureter, and bladder

KUS
    kidney, ureter and spleen

KV
    killed vaccine

kV
    kilovolt

kVa
    kilovolt-ampere

KVO
    keep vein open

kVp
    kilovolts peak

KW
    Keith-Wagener (test)
    Kimmelstiel-Wilson
        (syndrome)

kW
    kilowatt

KWB
    Keith, Wagener, Barker

kx
    crystallography unit

kW-hr
    kilowatt-hour

L

coefficient of induction
lambert
left
length
lethal
ligament
light
light chain (of
  immunoglobulins)
lingual
liter
liver
lumbar
lumbar vertebra (L1–L5)
lung

L.

L. libra (pound)

L

Lactobacillus
luminance
self-inductance

L_0

limes nul

L+

limes tod

L_+

limes tod

L-

levo-

l

liter
lyxose

l.

L. ligamentum (ligament)

l

length

l-

levorotatory (enantiomer)

λ

decay constant
homosexuality
one of the two types of
  immunoglobulin light
  chains
microliter (now μl)
wavelength

L0

limes nul

LA

lactic acid
latex agglutination
left anterior
left arm
left atrial
left atrium
left auricle
leucine aminopeptidase
linguoaxial
local anesthesia
long acting

L & A

light and accommodation
  (reaction of pupils)

La

lanthanum

LAA

leukocyte ascorbic acid

lab

laboratory

LAC

long-arm cast

Lac

lactose

LAD

lactic acid dehydrogenase
left anterior descending
  (coronary artery)
left axis deviation

LAD *(continued)*
   lymphocyte-activating
      determinant

LAE
   left atrial enlargement

LAF
   laminar air flow
   lymphocyte activating
      factor

LAG
   labiogingival
   lymphangiogram

Lag.
   L. lagena (a flask)

LAH
   lactalbumin hydrolysate
   left atrial hypertrophy
   left anterior hemiblock

LAHB
   left anterior hemiblock

LAI
   labioincisal

LAIT
   latex agglutination-
      inhibition test

LAL
   Limulus amebocyte lysate

LAM
   laminectomy

lam
   laminectomy

LAMB
   lentigines, atrial myxoma,
      mucocutaneous myxomas,
      and blue nevi

lami
   laminotomy

LANC
   long-arm navicular cast

LAO
   left anterior oblique

LAP
   left atrial pressure
   leucine aminopeptidase
   leukocyte alkaline
      phosphatase
   lyophilized anterior
      pituitary (tissue)

LAR
   left arm recumbent

LAS
   linear alkyl sulfonate
   long-arm splint

LASER
   light amplification by
      stimulated emission of
      radiation

LAT
   lateral

lat
   lateral

Lat. dol.
   L. lateri dolenti (to the
      painful side)

lat men
   lateral meniscectomy

LATS
   long-acting thyroid
      stimulator

LATS-p
   LATS protector

LAV
   lymphadenopathy-
      associated virus

lb
   L. libra (pound)

LBB
   left bundle branch

LBBB
left bundle branch block

LBCD
left border of cardiac
dullness

LBD
left border dullness

LBF
Lactobacillus bulgaricus
factor

LBH
length, breadth, height

LBI
low serum-bound iron

LBM
lean body mass

LBNP
lower-body negative
pressure

LBP
low back pain
low blood pressure

LBT
lupus band test

LBW
low birth weight

LBWI
low birth weight infant

LC
lethal concentration
lipid cytosomes
liquid chromatography

LC$_{50}$
median lethal
concentration

LCA
left coronary artery
leukocyte common antigen

LCAT
lecithin-cholesterol
acyltransferase

LCCME
Liaison Committee on
Continuing Medical
Education

LCCS
low cervical cesarean
section

LCD
liquor carbonis detergens

LCF
left circumflex (coronary
artery)

LCFA
long-chain fatty acid

LCGME
Liaison Committee on
Graduate Medical
Education

L chain
light chain

LCL
large cell lymphoma
Levinthal-Coles-Lillie
(bodies)
lymphocytic leukemia
lymphocytic
lymphosarcoma

LCM
left costal margin
lymphatic
choriomeningitis
lymphocytic
choriomeningitis

LCME
Liaison Committee on
Medical Education

LCMV
> lymphocytic choriomeningitis virus

LCP
> Legg-Calvé-Perthes (disease)

LCSG
> Lung Cancer Study Group

LCT
> liquid crystal thermogram
> liquid crystal thermography
> long-chain triglyceride
> lymphocyte cytotoxic test

LD
> labyrinthine defect
> lactate dehydrogenase
> lactic dehydrogenase
> left deltoid
> legionnaires' disease
> lethal dose
> light difference
> linguodistal
> living donor
> lymphocyte-defined
> lymphocyte-depleted Hodgkin's disease

LD$_{50}$
> median lethal dose

LD 100
> invariably lethal dose

LD$_{100}$
> invariably lethal dose

L-D
> Leishman-Donovan (bodies)

LD 50 time
> median lethal time

LDA
> left descending artery
> left dorsoanterior
> linear displacement analysis

LDD
> light-dark discrimination

LDDS
> local dentist

LDH
> lactate dehydrogenase

LDL
> low-density lipoprotein

LDL-C
> low density lipoprotein–cholesterol

LDLP
> low-density lipoprotein

LDP
> left dorsoposterior

LDR
> labor, delivery, recovery

LDRP
> labor, delivery, recovery, postpartum

LDUB
> long double upright brace

LDV
> lactic dehydrogenase virus

LE
> left eye
> leukocyte esterase
> leukoerythrogenetic
> lower extremity
> lupus erythematosus

LEA
> lower extremity amputation

LE cell
> lupus erythematosus cell

LED
> lupus erythematosus disseminatus

Leg
    leg amputation

LEOPARD
    lentigines (multiple),
        electrocardiographic
        abnormalities, ocular
        hypertelorism,
        pulmonary stenosis,
        abnormalities of
        genitalia, retardation of
        growth, and
        sensorineural deafness

LE prep
    lupus erythematosus
        preparation

LES
    lower esophageal sphincter
    lupus erythematosus,
        systemic

les
    local excitatory state

LET
    linear energy transfer

LETS
    large, external
        transformation-sensitive
        fibronectin

Leu
    leucine

Leu-CAM
    leukocyte adhesion
        molecule

LF
    laryngofissure
    low forceps

Lf
    limit flocculation

LFA
    left femoral artery
    left forearm
    left frontoanterior

LFD
    lactose-free diet
    low-fat diet
    low forceps delivery

LFN
    lactoferrin

LFP
    left frontoposterior

LFT
    latex flocculation test
    left frontotransverse
    liver function test

LG
    large
    laryngectomy
    left gluteal
    linguogingival
    lymphography

LGA
    large for gestational age

LGB
    Landry-Guillain-Barré
        (syndrome)

LGB disease
    Landry-Guillain-Barré
        disease

LGL
    Lown-Ganong-Levine
        (syndrome)

LGN
    lateral geniculate nucleus
    lobular glomerulonephritis

LGV
    lymphogranuloma
        venereum

LH
    left hand
    left hyperphoria
    luteinizing hormone

LHF
    left heart failure

LH/FSH-RF
luteinizing hormone/follicle-stimulating hormone–releasing factor

LHL
left hepatic lobe

LHON
Leber's hereditary optic neuropathy

LH-RF
luteinizing hormone releasing factor

LH-RH
luteinizing hormone releasing hormone

LHT
left hypertropia

LHV
lymphotropic human herpesvirus

LI
linguoincisal

Li
lithium

LIA
leukemia-associated inhibitory activity

LIAFI
late infantile amaurotic familial idiocy

LIB
left in bottle

LIBC
latent iron-binding capacity

LIC
limiting isorrheic concentration

LICM
left intercostal margin

LI$_2$CO$_3$
lithium carbonate

LICS
left intercostal space

LIF
left iliac fossa
leukocyte inhibitory factor

lig.
ligament
ligamentum

ligg.
ligamenta
ligaments

LIH
left inguinal hernia

LIHA
low impulsiveness, high anxiety

LILA
low impulsiveness, low anxiety

LiMB
Listing of Molecular Biology Databases

LIQ
liquid
liquor
lower inner quadrant

Liq.
liquor

LIR
left iliac region

LIS
laboratory information system
left intercostal space
lobular in situ

LIV
left innominate vein

LIVIM
lethal intestinal virus of infant mice

LJM
Löwenstein-Jensen medium

LK
left kidney

Lkc
leukocyte

Lkcs
leukocytes

LKS
liver, kidneys, spleen

LL
left leg
left lower
left lung
lower lid
lower lobe
lysolecithin

LLB
long leg brace

LLC
liquid-liquid chromatography
long-leg cast

LLD
leg length discrepancy

LLD factor
Lactobacillus lactis Dorner factor

LLE
left lower extremity

LLF
Laki-Lorand factor

LLL
left lower leg
left lower limb
left lower lobe (of the lung)
left lower lung

LLM
localized leukocyte mobilization

LLQ
left lower quadrant

LLR
left lumbar region

LLS
lazy leukocyte syndrome
long-leg splint

LLWC
long-leg walking cast

LM
light microscopy
light minimum
linguomesial

lm
lumen

LMA
left mentoanterior

LMCA
left middle cerebral artery

LMD
local medical doctor
low molecular weight dextran

LME
left mediolateral episiotomy

LMF
lymphocyte mitogenic factor

LMM
lentigo maligna melanoma

LMP
last menstrual period
left mentoposterior

LMR
localized magnetic resonance

LMT
  left mentotransverse

LMW
  low molecular weight

LMWD
  low molecular weight
  dextran

LN
  lipoid nephrosis
  lupus nephritis
  lymph node

ln
  natural logarithm

LNMP
  last normal menstrual
  period

LNPF
  lymph node permeability
  factor

LO
  linguo-occlusal

LOA
  leave of absence
  left occipitoanterior

LOC
  level of consciousness
  location
  loss of consciousness

loc cit
  L. loco citato (in the place
  cited)

Loc. dol.
  L. loco dolenti (to the
  painful spot)

LOCS
  lens opacities classification
  system

LOD
  line of duty

log
  logarithm

loi
  limit of impurities

LOL
  left occipitolateral

LOM
  left otitis media
  limitation of motion
  loss of motion

LOMSA
  left otitis media,
  suppurative acute

LOMSC
  left otitis media,
  suppurative chronic

LOMSCh
  left otitis media,
  suppurative chronic

LOP
  left occipitoposterior

LOPP
  chlorambucil, vincristine,
  procarbazine, prednisone

LOQ
  lower outer quadrant

LOS
  length of stay

LOT
  left occipitotransverse

Lot.
  L. lotio (lotion)

LP
  latency period
  leukocyte-poor
  light perception
  linguopulpal
  lipoprotein
  low protein
  lumbar puncture
  lymphocyte-predominant
    Hodgkin's disease
  lymphoid plasma

L/P
   lactate-pyruvate ratio

LPA
   latex particle agglutination
   left pulmonary artery

Lp(a)
   lipoprotein little A antigen

L-PAM
   melphalan
      (L-phenylalanine
      mustard)

LPC
   late positive component

LPE
   lipoprotein electrophoresis

LPF
   leukocytosis-promoting
      factor
   localized plaque formation
   low-power field
   lymphocytosis-promoting
      factor

LPG
   liquefied propane gas

LPH
   left posterior hemiblock
   lipotropic hormone

LPHB
   left posterior hemiblock

LPL
   lipoprotein lipase

LPM
   liters per minute

lpm
   liters per minute

LPN
   licensed practical nurse

LPO
   left posterior oblique
   light perception only

LPS
   lipopolysaccharide

LPV
   left pulmonary veins

LQ
   lower quadrant

LR
   labor room
   laboratory references
   lactated Ringer's injection
   lactated Ringer's solution
   lateral rectus
   light reaction
   light reflex
   light-resistant

L/R
   left to right ratio

L&R
   left and right

L→R
   left to right

Lr
   lawrencium

LRCP
   Licentiate of the Royal
      College of Physicians

LRCP(E)
   Licentiate of the Royal
      College of Physicians
      (Edinburgh)

LRCP(I)
   Licentiate of the Royal
      College of Physicians
      (Ireland)

LRCS
   Licentiate of the Royal
      College of Surgeons

LRCS(E)
   Licentiate of the Royal
      College of Surgeons
      (Edinburgh)

LRCS(I)
Licentiate of the Royal College of Surgeons (Ireland)

LRD
local regional disease

LRF
luteinizing hormone releasing factor

LRFPS
Licentiate of the Royal Faculty of Physicians and Surgeons, a Scottish institution

LRH
luteinizing hormone releasing hormone

LRM
left radical mastectomy

LRQ
lower right quadrant

LRS
lactated Ringer's solution

LRT
lower respiratory tract

LS
left side
legally separated
liver and spleen
lumbosacral
lymphosarcoma

L/S
lecithin/sphingomyelin (ratio, in amniotic fluid)

LSA
left sacroanterior
Licentiate of Society of Apothecaries
lymphosarcoma

LSA_2-L_2
cyclophosphamide, vincristine, prednisone,

LSA_2-L_2
daunorubicin, methotrexate, cytarabine, thioguanine, olaspase, hydroxyurea, carmustine

LSA/RCS
lymphosarcoma–reticulum cell sarcoma

LSB
left sternal border

LSC
liquid-solid chromatography

LScA
left scapuloanterior

LScP
left scapuloposterior

LSCS
lower segment cesarean section

LSD
Letterer-Siwe disease
lumpy skin diseases virus
lysergic acid diethylamide

LSH
lutein-stimulating hormone
lymphocyte-stimulating hormone

LSI
large-scale integration

LSK
liver, spleen, and kidneys

LSL
left sacrolateral

LSM
late systolic murmur

LSO
lumbosacral orthosis

LSP
left sacroposterior

L-sp
  lumbar spine

L-spine
  lumbar spine

L-S ratio
  lecithin-syringomyelin
    ratio (in amniotic fluid)

LST
  left sacrotransverse

LSV
  left subclavian vein

LT
  left
  left thigh
  Levin tube
  levothyroxine
  L-tryptophan
  lung transplantation
  lymphotoxin

LTA
  lipoteichoic acid

LTB
  laryngotracheobronchitis

LTB$_4$, LTC$_4$
  symbols for various
    leukotrienes

LTC
  long term care

LTCP
  L-tryptophan–containing
    products

LTF
  lymphocyte transforming
    factor

LTH
  lactogenic hormone
  luteotropic hormone

lt lat
  left lateral

LTM
  long-term memory

LTPP
  lipothiamide
    pyrophosphate

LTR
  long terminal repeat

LTT
  lymphoblastic
    transformation test
  lymphocyte transformation
    test

LU
  left upper

L&U
  lower and upper

Lu
  lutetium

LUE
  left upper extremity

Lues I
  primary syphilis

Lues II
  secondary syphilis

Lues III
  tertiary syphilis

LUL
  left upper limb
  left upper lobe (of lungs)
  left upper lung

lumb
  lumbar

LUOQ
  left upper outer quadrant

LUQ
  left upper quadrant

LV
  left ventricle
  leukemia virus
  leukovorin
  live virus

Lv
>   leukovorin

LVB
>   lomustine, vindesine, and
>   bleomycin sulfate

LVDP
>   left ventricular diastolic
>   pressure

LVDV
>   left ventricular diastolic
>   volume

LVE
>   left ventricular ejection
>   left ventricular
>   enlargement

LVEDP
>   left ventricular
>   end-diastolic pressure

LVEDV
>   left ventricular
>   end-diastolic volume

LVEP
>   left ventricular
>   end-pressure

LVET
>   left ventricular ejection
>   time

LVF
>   left ventricular failure
>   low-voltage fast
>   low-voltage foci

LVH
>   large vessel hematocrit
>   left ventricular
>   hypertrophy

LVN
>   licensed vocational nurse
>   Licensed Visiting Nurse

LVP
>   left ventricular pressure
>   lysine vasopressin

LVS
>   left ventricular strain

LVSP
>   left ventricular systolic
>   pressure

LVSV
>   left ventricular stroke
>   volume

LVSW
>   left ventricular stroke
>   work

LVW
>   left ventricular wall
>   left ventricular work

LVWI
>   left ventricular work index

LW
>   Lee-White (method)

L&W
>   living and well

LX
>   local irradiation

lx
>   lux

lymphs
>   lymphocytes

Lys
>   lysine

lytes
>   electrolytes

Lyx
>   lyxose

lzm
>   lysozyme

M
macerate
male
married
mass
maternal
maximal
mechlorethamine
  hydrochloride
mega-
meter
minim
molar
moles per liter
morgan
mother
mucoid (colony)
multipara
murmur
muscle
myopia
permanent molar
strength of pole
thousand

M.
L. misce (mix)
L. mistura (mixture)

M
molar (concentration)
molar mass
mutual inductance

M.
Micrococcus
Microsporum
Mycobacterium
Mycoplasma

M_1
mitral valve closure

M_L
left electrode

M_R
right electrode

M_r
relative molecular weight

M_r
relative molecular mass

M/3
middle third

M1
matrix protein 1

M2
matrix protein 2

Ⓜ
murmur

m
married
median
meter
milli-

m.
minim
L. musculus (muscle)

m
mass
molal

m-
meta-

μ
electrophoretic mobility
the heavy chain of IgM
linear attenuation
  coefficient
mass absorption coefficient
micro-
micron
population mean

MA
mandelic acid
Master of Arts
mean arterial (blood
  pressure)

MA *(continued)*
    menstrual age
    mental age
    meter angle
    Miller-Abbott (tube)

Ma
    masurium

mA
    milliampere

μA
    microampere

MAA
    macroaggregated albumin

mAB
    monoclonal antibody

MABOP
    mechlorethamine,
    doxorubicin, bleomycin
    sulfate, vincristine, and
    prednisone

MABP
    mean arterial blood
    pressure

MAC
    maximum allowable
    concentration
    membrane attack complex
    methotrexate,
    dactinomycin,
    chlorambucil
    minimal alveolar
    concentration

Mac.
    L. macerare (macerate)

MACC
    methotrexate, doxorubicin,
    cyclophosphamide,
    lomustine

MAC INH
    membrane attack complex
    inhibitor

MACOP-B
    methotrexate, doxorubicin,
    cyclophosphamide,
    vincristine, prednisone,
    bleomycin, cotrimoxazole

MACP
    Master of the American
    College of Physicians

MAD
    maximal acid output

MADD
    multiple acyl CoA
    dehydrogenation
    deficiency

MAE
    moves all extremities

MAF
    macrophage activating
    factor

MAFH
    macroaggregated ferrous
    hydroxide

Mag.
    L. magnus (large)

mag. cit.
    magnesium citrate

MAggF
    macrophage agglutination
    factor

MAHA
    microangiopathic
    hemolytic aneurysm

MAKA
    major karyotypic
    abnormalities

MAL
    midaxillary line

malig
    malignant

MAM
methylazomethanol

M + Am
myopic astigmatism

Man.
L. manipulus (a handful)
mannose

manifest
manifestation

Manip.
L. manipulus (a handful)

MANOVA
multivariate analysis of
variance

Man. pr.
L. mane primo (early in
the morning)

MAO
maximum acid output
monoamine oxidase

MAOI
monoamine oxidase
inhibitor

MAP
mean aortic pressure
mean arterial pressure
megaloblastic anemia of
pregnancy
methylacetoxyprogesterone
methylaminopurine
muscle-action potential

MAPF
microatomized protein food

mAs
milliampere-seconds

mas
milliampere-second

masc
mass concentration

MASER
microwave amplification
by stimulated emission of
radiation
molecular application by
stimulated emission of
radiation

MASH
mobile army surgical unit

Mas. pil.
L. massa pilularum (pill
mass)

massc
mass concentration

massfr
mass fraction

mass spec
mass spectrometry

MAST
military (medical)
anti-shock trousers

MAT
multifocal atrial
tachycardia

Matut.
L. matutinus (in the
morning)

MAVIS
mobile artery and vein
imaging system

max
maximum

MB
buccal margin
L. Medicinae Baccalaureus
(Bachelor of Medicine)
mesiobuccal
methylene blue
microbiological assay

Mb
myoglobin

m.b.
L. misce bene (mix well)

MBA
methylbovine albumin

M-BACOD
methotrexate, bleomycin, doxorubicin, cyclophosphamide, vincristine, dexamethasone

MBAS
methylene blue active substance

MBC
maximum breathing capacity
minimal bactericidal concentration

MbCO
myoglobin combined with carbon monoxide

MBD
methotrexate, bleomycin, cisplatin
methylene blue dye
minimal brain damage
minimal brain dysfunction
Morquio-Brailsford disease

MBF
myocardial blood flow

MBK
methyl butyl ketone

MBL
menstrual blood loss
minimal bactericidal level

MBO
mesiobucco-occlusal

MbO$_2$
myoglobin combined with oxygen

MBP
mean blood pressure
melitensis, bovine, porcine (antigen prepared from *Brucella melitensis, B. bovis,* and *B. suis*)
mesiobuccopulpal
myelin basic protein

MBq
megabecquerel

MBSA
methylated bovine serum albumin

MC
L. Magister Chirurgiae (Master of Surgery)
mast cell
maximum concentration
Medical Corps
metacarpal
metacarpal amputation
mineralocorticoid
mitomycin-C
mixed-cellularity Hodgkin's disease
myocarditis

MC 540
merocyanine 540

M&C
morphine and cocaine

Mc
megacurie
megacycle

mC
millicoulomb

mc
former abbreviation for millicurie

m+c
morphine and cocaine

μC
microcoulomb

MCA
  Manufacturing Chemists
    Association
  3-methylcholanthrene
  middle cerebral artery
  multichannel analyzer

MCAT
  Medical College Admission
    Test

MCB
  membranous cytoplasmic
    body

MCBR
  minimum concentration of
    bilirubin

MCC
  mean corpuscular
    hemoglobin concentration
  minimum complete-killing
    concentration

MCCU
  mobile coronary care unit

MCD
  mean cell diameter
  mean of consecutive
    differences
  mean corpuscular diameter
  medullary cystic disease

MCF
  African malignant
    catarrhal fever
  macrophage chemotactic
    factor
  mitoxantrone,
    cyclophosphamide,
    fluorouracil

MCFA
  medium-chain fatty acid

Mcg
  an immunoglobulin λlight
    chain antigenic marker

mcg
  microgram

MCH
  mean corpuscular
    hemoglobin

mch
  millicurie-hour

MCHB
  Maternal and Child Health
    Bureau

MCHC
  mean corpuscular
    hemoglobin concentration

MCHg
  mean corpuscular
    hemoglobin

MCI
  mean cardiac index

MCi
  megacurie

mCi
  millicurie

μCi
  microcurie

mCi-hr
  millicurie-hour

μCi-hr
  microcurie-hour

MCL
  midclavicular line
  midcostal line
  modified chest lead
  most comfortable loudness
    level

MCMI
  Millon clinical multiaxial
    inventory

MCP
  metacarpophalangeal
  mitotic-control protein

Mcps
  megacycles per second

MCR
steroid metabolic clearance
rate

M-CSF
macrophage
colony-stimulating factor

MCT
mean cell threshold
mean circulation time
mean corpuscular
thickness
medium-chain triglyceride
medullary carcinoma of
the thyroid

MCTD
mixed connective tissue
disease

MCV
mean corpuscular volume

MD
malic dehydrogenase
manic-depressive
Mantoux diameter
Marek's disease
L. Medicinae Doctor
(Doctor of Medicine)
mediodorsal
mesiodistal
movement disorder
muscular dystrophy
myocardial damage
myocardial disease

Md
mendelevium

MDA
M.D. Anderson Hospital
and Tumor Institute
L. mentodextra anterior
(right mentoanterior)
methylenedioxyamphet-
amine
motor discriminative
acuity

MDC
minimum detectable
concentration

MDF
mean dominant frequency
myocardial depressant
factor

MDH
malate dehydrogenase
malic dehydrogenase

MDI
manic-depressive illness

M. Dict.
L. more dicto (as directed)

MDM
minor determinant
mixture (of penicillin)

MDP
L. mentodextra posterior
(right mentoposterior)
methylene diphosphonate

MDR
minimum daily
requirement

M.D.S.
Master of Dental Surgery

MDT
median detection threshold
mentodextra transversa
(right mentotransverse)

MDTR
mean diameter-thickness
ratio

MDUO
myocardial disease of
unknown origin

MDY
month, date, year

ME
medical examiner

ME *(continued)*
  mercaptoethanol
  middle ear

M/E
  myeloid-erythroid (ratio)

Me
  methyl

MEA
  mercaptoethylamine
  multiple endocrine
    abnormalities
  multiple endocrine
    adenomatosis
  multiple endocrine
    adenopathies

MEC
  minimum effective
    concentration
  meconium

mec
  meconium

MeCbl
  methylcobalamin

MeCCNU
  semustine

MeCcnu
  semustine

Me₂CO
  acetone

MED
  median erythrocyte
    diameter
  minimal effective dose
  minimal erythema dose

med
  medial
  medical
  medicine

MEDAC
  multiple endocrine
    deficiency–Addison's
    disease–candidiasis

MEDLARS
  Medical Literature
    Analysis and Retrieval
    System

MEDLINE
  MEDLARS-on-line

MEF
  maximal expiratory flow

MEFR
  maximal expiratory flow
    rate

MEFV
  maximal expiratory flow
    volume

MEG
  magnetoencephalogram
  magnetoencephalograph
  magnetoencephalography
  megakaryocytes
  megestrol acetate

Meg
  megestrol acetate

Meg-CSF
  megakaryocytic
    colony-stimulating factor

MEGX
  monoethylglycinexylidide

MEI
  Medicare Economic Index

MEK
  methyl ethyl ketone

MEM
  minimum essential
    medium

MEN
  multiple endocrine
    neoplasia

MeOH
  methyl alcohol

MEP
    motor evoked potential
    multimodality evoked
        potential

MEPP
    miniature end-plate
        potential

mEq
    milliequivalent

meq
    milliequivalent

mEq/L
    milliequivalents per liter

MER
    mean ejection rate
    methanol extraction
        residue

MER-29
    triparanol

MET
    metabolic equivalent

Met
    methionine

metab
    metabolism
    metabolites

metHb
    methemoglobin

metMb
    metmyoglobin

mets
    metastases

M. et sig.
    L. misce et signa (mix and
        write a label)

MEV
    million electron volts

MeV
    megaelectron volt
    million electron volts

Mev
    megaelectron volt

meV
    millielectron volt

mev
    million electron volts

MF
    medium frequency
    microscopic factor
    mycosis fungoides
    myelin figures

M&F
    mother and father

mF
    millifarad

mf
    microfilaria

μF
    microfarad

MFB
    metallic foreign body

MFD
    midforceps delivery
    minimal fatal dose

mfg
    manufacturing

M. flac.
    L. membrana flaccida (pars
        flaccida membranae
        tympani)

MFP
    monofluorophosphate

MFR
    mucus flow rate

mfr
    manufacture

MFT
    muscle function test

M. ft.
> L. mistura fiat (let a
> mixture be made)

MG
> menopausal gonadotropin
> mesiogingival
> methyl glucoside
> muscle group
> myasthenia gravis

Mg
> magnesium

mg
> milligram

mg %
> milligrams per 100
> milliliters

mγ
> milligamma (nanogram)

μg
> microgram

$\mu\gamma$
> microgamma (picogram)

MGB
> Michaelis-Gutmann bodies

MGBG
> methylglyoxal
> *bis*(guanylhydrazone)

MGF
> maternal grandfather

MGGH
> methylglyoxal
> guanylhydrazone

mgh
> milligram-hour

MGM
> maternal grandmother

mgm
> milligram

MGN
> membranous
> glomerulonephritis

MgO
> magnesium oxide

MGP
> marginal granulocyte pool

MGR
> modified gain ratio

MgSO$_4$
> magnesium sulfate

mgtis
> meningitis

MGUS
> monoclonal gammopathy
> of undetermined
> significance

MH
> mammotropic hormone
> marital history
> menstrual history
> mental health

mH
> millihenry

MHA
> methemalbumin
> microangiopathic
> hemolytic anemia
> microhemagglutination
> mixed hemadsorption

MHA-TP
> microhemagglutination
> assay–*Treponema
> pallidum*

MHB
> maximum hospital benefit

MHb
> methemoglobin

MHC
> major histocompatibility
> complex

MHD
> mean hemolytic dose
> minimum hemolytic dose

mHg
> millimeters of mercury

MHN
> massive hepatic necrosis

MHP
> 1-mercuri-2-hydroxy-
> propane

MHPG
> methoxyhydroxyphenyl-
> glycol

MHR
> maximal heart rate

MHW
> medial heel wedge

MHz
> megahertz

MI
> mercaptoimidazole
> mitral incompetence
> mitral insufficiency
> myocardial infarction

MIBG
> metaiodobenzylguanidine

MIBI
> sestamibi

MIBK
> methyl isobutyl ketone

MIC
> maternal and infant care
> minimal inhibitory
> concentration
> minimal isorrheic
> concentration

microcryst
> microcrystalline

MICU
> medical intensive care unit
> mobile intensive care unit

MID
> maximum inhibiting
> dilution
> mesioincisodistal
> minimum infective dose
> minimum inhibiting dose

middle/3
> middle third

MIF
> macrophage-inhibiting
> factor
> melanocyte-stimulating
> hormone inhibiting factor
> migration inhibiting factor
> mixed immunofluorescence

MIFR
> maximal inspiratory flow
> rate

MIME
> methyl GAG, ifosfamide,
> methotrexate, and
> etoposide

min
> mineral
> minor
> minute

min.
> L. minimum (minim)

MIO
> minimal identifiable odor

MIP
> maximum inspiratory
> pressure

MIPS
> Martinsreid Institute for
> Protein Sequence

MIRD
> Medical Internal Radiation
> Dose

MIS
> minimal intervention
> surgery

MIS *(continued)*
    müllerian inhibiting
        substance

misc
    miscarriage
    miscellaneous
    miscible

mist.
    L. mistura (mixture)

MIT
    monoiodotyrosine

Mit.
    L. mitte (send)

MIU
    milli-international unit

mixt
    mixture

MJ
    marijuana

MK
    monkey lung (cell culture)
    monkey kidney
    menaquinone

MK-6
    menaquinone-6

MK-7
    menaquinone-7

MKS
    meter-kilogram-second

mks
    meter-kilogram-second

MKV
    killed-measles vaccine

ML
    mesiolingual
    middle lobe
    midline

M/L
    monocyte to lymphocyte
        (ratio)

mL
    millilambert

ml
    milliliter

μl
    microliter

MLA
    L. mentolaeva anterior
        (left mentoanterior)
    Medical Library
        Association
    mesiolabial
    monocytic leukemia, acute

MLAI
    mesiolabioincisal

MLAP
    mean left atrial pressure

MLBW
    moderately low birth
        weight

MLC
    minimum lethal
        concentration
    mixed leukocyte culture
    mixed lymphocyte culture
    multilamellar cytosome
    myelomonocytic leukemia,
        chronic

MLD
    median lethal dose
    metachromatic
        leukodystrophy
    minimum lethal dose

MLI
    mesiolinguoincisal

MLMV
    Medical Lake macaque
        virus

MLNS
    mucocutaneous lymph
        node syndrome

MLO
>   mesiolinguo-occlusal

MLP
>   L. mentolaeva posterior
>   (left mentoposterior)
>   mesiolinguopulpal

MLR
>   mixed lymphocyte reaction

MLS
>   myelomonocytic leukemia,
>   subacute

MLT
>   L. mentolaeva transversa
>   (left mentotransverse)

MLV
>   Moloney's leukemogenic
>   virus
>   mouse leukemia virus

MM
>   malignant melanoma
>   Marshall-Marchetti
>   (procedure)
>   medial malleolus
>   mucous membranes
>   multiple myeloma
>   muscles
>   muscularis mucosa
>   myeloid metaplasia

M&M
>   milk and molasses

mM
>   millimolar
>   millimole

mm
>   millimeter
>   mucous membrane

mμ
>   millimicron

μM
>   micromolar

μm
>   micrometer

$\mu\mu$
>   micromicro-

MMA
>   methylmalonic acid
>   monocyte monolayer assay

MMC
>   minimal medullary
>   concentration

MMC C
>   mitomycin C

Mmc C
>   mitomycin C

mμCi
>   millimicrocurie (nanocurie)

$\mu\mu$Ci
>   micromicrocurie (picocurie)

MMD
>   minimal morbidostatic
>   dose

MMEF
>   maximum midexpiratory
>   flow

MMEFR
>   maximum midexpiratory
>   flow rate

MMF
>   maximum midexpiratory
>   flow

MMFR
>   maximum midexpiratory
>   flow rate
>   maximum midflow rate

mμg
>   millimicrogram
>   (nanogram)

μmg
>   micromilligram

$\mu\mu$g
>   micromicrogram
>   (picogram)

mm Hg
 millimeters of mercury

MMIHS
 megacystis-microcolon–
  intestinal hypoperistalsis
  syndrome

mM/L
 millimoles per liter

mM/l
 millimoles per liter

MMM
 myelofibrosis with myeloid
  metaplasia
 myelosclerosis with
  myeloid metaplasia

μmm
 micromillimeter

mmol
 millimole

mmp
 mixture melting point

MMPI
 Minnesota Multiphasic
  Personality Inventory

mmpp
 millimeters partial
  pressure

MMPR
 methylmercaptopurine
  roboside

MMR
 mass miniature
  radiography
 measles-mumps-rubella
  (vaccine)
 myocardial metabolic rate

MMRV
 measles-mumps-rubella-
  varicella

MMS
 Massachusetts Medical
  Society

MMT
 manual muscle test

MMTV
 mouse mammary tumor
  virus

MMWR
 Morbidity and Mortality
  Weekly Report

MN
 midnight
 motor neuron
 multinodular
 myoneural

M&N
 morning and night

Mn
 manganese

mN
 millinormal

MNCV
 motor nerve conduction
  velocity

MnPV
 Mastomys natalensis
  papillomavirus

MNSs
 blood group

MNU
 methylnitrosourea

MO
 Medical Officer
 mesio-occlusal
 mineral oil

Mo
 molybdenum
 month
 mother
 mouth

mo
> month
> mother
> motor

MOAB
> monoclonal antibody

MOCA
> methotrexate, vincristine, cyclophosphamide, and doxorubicin

MOD
> mesio-occlusodistal
> moderate

MODM
> mature-onset diabetes mellitus

Mod. praesc.
> L. modo praescripto (in the way directed)

MODY
> maturity-onset diabetes of youth

MOF
> 5-fluorouracil, methylCCNU, and vincristine

mol
> mole

molal.
> molality

molc
> molar concentration

Mol wt
> molecular weight

MOM
> milk of magnesia

MOMA
> methoxyhydroxymandelic acid

mono
> infectious mononucleosis

MOP
> mechlorethamine, vincristine, procarbazine

8-MOP
> 8-methoxypsoralen

MOPLACE
> cyclophosphamide, etoposide, prednisone, methotrexate, cytarabine, and vincristine

MOPP
> mechlorethamine, vincristine, procarbazine, and prednisone

MOPP/ABVD
> mechlorethamine hydrochloride, vincristine, procarbazine, prednisone, doxorubicin, bleomycin, vinblastine, and dacarbazine

MOPV
> monovalent oral poliovirus vaccine

MORC
> Medical Officers Reserve Corps

Mor. dict.
> L. more dicto (in the manner directed)

Mor. sol.
> L. more solito (in the usual way)

mOs
> milliosmolal

mOsm
> milliosmole

MOTT
> mycobacteria other than tubercle bacilli

MP

mean pressure
melting point
menstrual period
mercaptopurine
mesiopulpal
metacarpophalangeal
metaphalangeal
metatarsophalangeal
methylprednisolone
mononuclear phagocyte
monophosphate
mucopolysaccharide
multiparous

6-MP

6-mercaptopurine

Mp

6-mercaptopurine

mp

melting point

m.p.

L. modo prescripto (as
directed)

MPA

main pulmonary artery
mantle-paraaortic-splenic
(irradiation)
medroxyprogesterone
acetate
methylprednisolone
acetate

MPAP

mean pulmonary arterial
pressure

MPAS

mantle-paraaortic-splenic
(irradiation)

MPC

marine protein concentrate
maximum permissible
concentration
meperidine, promethazine,
chlorpromazine

MPC *(continued)*

minimum
mycoplasmacidal
concentration
mucopurulent cervicitis

MPD

maximum permissible dose

MPEH

methylphenylethyl-
hydantoin

MPGN

membranoproliferative
glomerulonephritis

MPH

Master of Public Health

MPI

multiphasic personality
inventory

MPJ

metacarpophalangeal joint

MPL

maximum permissible
level
mesiopulpolingual

MPO

myeloperoxidase

MPP

mercaptopyrazido-
pyrimidine

mppcf

millions of particles per
cubic foot

MPPP

1-methyl-4-phenyl-4-propion-
oxypiperidine

MPS

mononuclear phagocyte
system
mucopolysaccharides
mucopolysaccharidosis
multiphasic screening

MPV
metatarsus primus varus

MQ
former abbreviation for menaquinone

MR
magnetic resonance
medial rectus
medical report
megaroentgen
mental retardation
metabolic rate
methyl red
mitral reflux
mitral regurgitation
mortality rate
mortality ratio
motor retardation
muscle relaxant

M&R
measure and record

mR
milliroentgen

μR
microroentgen

MRA
Medical Record Administrator

MRACP
Member of Royal Australasian College of Physicians

mrad
millirad

MRAP
mean right atrial pressure

MRC
Medical Research Council of Great Britain
Medical Reserve Corps

MRCP
Member of the Royal College of Physicians

MRCPE
Member of the Royal College of Physicians of Edinburgh

MRCP (Glasg)
Member of the Royal College of Physicians and Surgeons of Glasgow qua Physician

MRCPI
Member of the Royal College of Physicians of Ireland

MRCS
Member of the Royal College of Surgeons

MRCSE
Member of the Royal College of Surgeons of Edinburgh

MRCSI
Member of the Royal College of Surgeons of Ireland

MRCVS
Member of the Royal College of Veterinary Surgeons

MRD
minimum reacting dose

mrem
millirem

MRF
melanocyte-stimulating hormone releasing factor
mesencephalic reticular formation
mitral regurgitant flow

MRFIT
Multiple Risk Factor Intervention Trial

MRI
> magnetic resonance
> imaging

MRL
> Medical Record Librarian
> (now Medical Record
> Administrator)

mRNA
> messenger RNA

MRSA
> methicillin-resistant
> *Staphylococcus aureus*

MRVP
> mean right ventricular
> pressure

MS
> mass spectrometry
> Master of Surgery
> mental status
> mitral stenosis
> morphine sulfate
> mucosubstance
> multiple sclerosis
> muscle strength
> musculoskeletal

ms
> millisecond

μs
> microsecond

MSA
> multiplication-stimulating
> activity

MSB
> most significant bit

MSBOS
> maximal surgical blood
> order schedule

MSc
> Master of Science

MSD
> Master of Science in
> Dentistry

MSD *(continued)*
> Merck Sharp & Dohme, Inc
> most significant digit

msec
> millisecond

μsec
> microsecond

MSER
> mean systolic ejection rate

MSG
> monosodium glutamate

MSH
> melanocyte-stimulating
> hormone
> melanophore-stimulating
> hormone

MSH-IF
> melanocyte-stimulating
> hormone inhibiting factor

MSH-RF
> melanocyte-stimulating
> hormone releasing factor

MSK
> medullary sponge kidney

MSKCC
> Memorial Sloan-Kettering
> Cancer Center

MSL
> midsternal line

MSLA
> mouse-specific lymphocyte
> antigen

MSN
> Master of Science in
> Nursing

MSSA
> methicillin-susceptible
> *Staphylococcus aureus*

MSSU
> mid-stream specimen of
> urine

MST
mean survival time
median graft survival time

MsTh$_1$
mesothorium-1

MsTh$_2$
mesothorium-2

MSU
midstream urine
(specimen)
monosodium urate

MSUD
maple syrup urine disease

MSV
Moloney's sarcoma virus
murine sarcoma virus

MSW
Master of Social Work

MT
empty
malignant teratoma
Medical Technologist
Medical Transcriptionist
membrana tympani
metatarsal
metatarsal amputation
methyltyrosine
muscles and tendons
music therapy

MTA
metatarsus adductus

MT bar
metatarsal bar

MTBF
mean time between
failures

MTC
medullary thyroid
carcinoma
minimum toxic
concentration

MTCA
1-methyl-1,2,3,4-tetrahydro-
β-carboline-3-carboxylic
acid

MTD
maximally tolerated dose

mtDNA
mitochondrial
deoxyribonucleic acid

MTF
maximum terminal flow
modulation transfer
function

MTHF
methyltetrahydrofolic acid

MTI
malignant teratoma,
intermediate

MTJ
midtarsal joint

MTP
metatarsophalangeal

MTR
mean total reactivity
Meinicke turbidity
reaction

MTT
malignant trophoblastic
teratoma
monotetrazolium

MTU
methylthiouracil

MTV
mammary tumor virus
metatarsus varus

MTX
methotrexate

Mtx
methotrexate

MTX-CHOP
  methotrexate,
    cyclophosphamide,
    doxorubicin, vincristine,
    and prednisone

MU
  Montevideo unit

Mu
  Mache unit

mU
  milliunit

mu
  micron

m.u.
  mouse unit

μU
  microunit

MUAP
  motor unit action potential

MUC
  maximum urinary
    concentration

Muc.
  L. mucilago (mucilage)

MUGA
  multiple gated acquisition

MUMPS
  Massachusetts
    Utility-Multi-Program-
    ming System

MUO
  metastasis of unknown
    origin

MUP
  motor unit potential

Mur
  muramic acid

musc
  muscles

musc *(continued)*
  muscular

MUST
  mechlorethamine
    hydrochloride
    (Mustargen)

Must
  mechlorethamine
    hydrochloride
    (Mustargen)

MUU
  mouse uterine units

MV
  L. Medicus Veterinarius
    (veterinary physician)
  megavolt
  minute volume
  mitral valve
  mixed venous

Mv
  mendelevium

mV
  millivolt

μV
  microvolt

MVA
  motor vehicle accident

MVM
  microvillose membrane

MVO_2
  myocardial oxygen
    ventilation rate

MVP
  mitral valve prolapse

MVPP
  mechlorethamine,
    vinblastine, procarbazine,
    prednisone

MVR
  massive vitreous retraction

MVV
maximum voluntary
ventilation

MW
molecular weight

mW
milliwatt

mw
microwave

μW
microwatt

MWD
microwave diathermy

Mx
maxwell
Medex

mx
management

My
myopia

my
mayer

MyG
myasthenia gravis

MZ
monozygotic

m/z
mass to charge ratio

N

nasal
negative
nerve
newton
nitrogen
normal (solution)
normal concentration
size of sample
unit of neutron dosage

N

Avogadro's number
Neisseria
neutron number
Nocardia
normal
number
population size

N_A

Avogadro's number

Ⓝ

notified

n

nano-
nausea
neutron
normal
refractive index

n.

L. nervus (nerve)

n

(haploid) chromosome
number
refractive index
sample size

n-

normal

n_D

refractive index

ν

degrees of freedom
frequency
kinematic viscosity
neutrino

NA

neuraminidase
neutralizing antibody
nicotinic acid
Nomina Anatomica
noradrenalin
not admitted
not applicable
not available
numerical aperture

N/A

not applicable

Na

sodium

NAA

neutron activation analysis
no apparent abnormalities

NAACLS

National Accrediting
Agency for Clinical
Laboratory Science

NAACOG

Nurses Association of the
American Association of
Obstetrics and
Gynecology

NaBr

sodium bromide

NABX

needle aspiration biopsy

NACA

National Advisory Council
on Aging

NAC-EDTA
    N-acetyl-L-cysteine
    ethylenediaminetetra-
    acetic acid

NaCl
    sodium chloride

NaClO
    sodium hypochlorite

NaClO$_3$
    sodium chlorate

NAcneu
    N-acetylneuraminic acid

Na$_2$CO$_3$
    sodium carbonate

Na$_2$C$_2$O$_4$
    sodium oxalate

NACT
    National Alliance of
    Cardiovascular
    Technologists

NAD
    nicotinamide-adenine
      dinucleotide
    no abnormality detected
    no active disease
    no acute distress
    no appreciable disease
    normal axis deviation
    nothing abnormal detected

NAD$^+$
    the oxidized form of NAD

NADH
    the reduced form of NAD
    methemoglobin reductase

NADL
    National Association of
    Dental Laboratories

NADONA/LTC
    National Association of
    Directors of Nursing in
    Long Term Care

NADP
    nicotinamide-adenine
    dinucleotide phosphate

NADP$^+$
    the oxidized form of NADP

NADPH
    the reduced form of NADP

NAEMT
    National Association of
    Emergency Medical
    Technicians

NAHC
    National Association for
    Home Care

NAHM
    National Association for
    Mental Health

NAHSR
    National Association of
    Human Services
    Technologists

NAI
    non-accidental injury

NAME
    nevi, atrial myxoma,
    myxoid neurofibromas,
    and ephilides

NAMT
    National Association for
    Music Therapy

NAN
    N- acetylneuraminic acid

Nan
    nitrosamine

NANA
    N-acetylneuraminic acid

NANBH
    non-A, non-B hepatitis

NANBV
    non-A, non-B virus

NANDA
North American Nursing
Diagnosis Association

NANPHR
National Association of
Nurse Practitioners in
Reproductive Health

NANSAIDS
nonaspirin, nonsteroidal,
anti-inflammatory drugs

NAP
nasion, point A, pogonion

NAPA
N-acetylated procainamide
N-acetyl-*p*-aminophenol

NAPNES
National Association for
Practical Nurse
Education and Services

NARF
National Association of
Rehabilitation Facilities

NAS
nasal
no added salt

NAS-NRC
National Academy of
Sciences–National
Research Council

NASW
National Association of
Social Workers

NAT
neonatal alloimmune
thrombocytopenia

nat
national

NATP
neonatal alloimmune
thrombocytopenia

NATTS
National Association of
Trade and Technical
Schools

NB
newborn
nitrous oxide-barbiturate
L. nota bene (note well)

Nb
niobium

NBCCGA
National Bladder Cancer
Collaborative Group A

NBI
no bone injury

NBM
nothing by mouth

NBME
National Board of Medical
Examiners

NBS
National Bureau of
Standards
normal blood serum

NBT
nitroblue tetrazolium

NBTE
nonbacterial thrombotic
endocarditis

NBTNF
newborn, term, normal,
female

NBTNM
newborn, term, normal,
male

NBW
normal birth weight

NC
no change
no complaints

NC *(continued)*
    noncontributory
    not cultured

NCA
    neurocirculatory asthenia
    nonspecific cross-reacting
        antigen

NCAMLP
    National Certification
        Agency for Medical
        Laboratory Personnel

NCBI
    National Center for
        Biotechnology
        Information

NCCLS
    National Committee for
        Clinical Laboratory
        Standards

NCCTG
    North Central Cancer
        Treatment Group

NCEHPHP
    National Council on the
        Education of Health
        Professionals in Health
        Promotion

NCF
    neutrophil chemotactic
        factor

NCHLS
    National Council of Health
        Laboratory Services

NCHS
    National Center Health
        Statistics

NCI
    National Cancer Institute

nCi
    nanocurie

NCMH
    National Committee
        Mental Hygiene

NCN
    National Council of Nurses

NCRE
    National Council on
        Rehabilitation Education

NCRP
    National Committee on
        Radiation Protection and
        Measurements

NCV
    nerve conduction velocity
    noncholera vibrios

ND
    natural death
    neonatal death
    Newcastle disease
    no disease
    nondisabling
    normal delivery
    not done

Nd
    neodymium

N_D
    refractive index

nd
    not done

NDA
    National Dental
        Association
    new drug application
    no data available
    no demonstrable antibodies

NDGA
    nordihydroguaiaretic acid

NDI
    nephrogenic diabetes
        insipidus

NDMA
nitrosodimethylaniline

NDMS
National Disaster Medical
System

NDP
net dietary protein
nucleoside 5′-phosphate

NDV
Newcastle disease virus

Nd:YAG
neodymium:yttrium-alumin-
um-garnet

NE
nerve ending
neurologic examination
no effect
nonelastic
norepinephrine
not enlarged
not examined

Ne
neon

NEC
necrotizing enterocolitis
not elsewhere classified

nec.
not elsewhere classified

NED
no evidence of disease

NEEP
negative end-expiratory
pressure

NEFA
nonesterified fatty acids

neg
negative

NEHA
National Environmental
Health Education

NEI
National Eye Institute

NEM
N-ethylmaleimide

NER
no evidence of recurrence

NERD
no evidence of recurrent
disease

NES
not elsewhere specified

net.
Network

neu
neuraminic acid

NF
National Formulary
none found
not found
not felt

nF
nanofarad

nf
not felt

NFLPN
National Federation for
Licensed Practical Nurses

NFTD
normal full term delivery

NG
nasogastric
no good

ng
millimicrogram
nanogram

NGF
nerve growth factor

ngm
nanogram

NGU
nongonococcal urethritis

NH
nodular histiocytic
lymphoma
nursing home

NH$_3$
ammonia

NHA
nonspecific hepatocellular
abnormality

NHANES-I
National Health and
Nutrition Examination
Survey I

NHC
National Health Council
neonatal hypocalcemia
nonhistone chromosomal
(protein)

NHEFS
NHANES Epidemiologic
Followup Study

NHIS
National Health Interview
Survey

NHL
nodular histiocytic
lymphoma
non-Hodgkin's lymphoma

NHLBI
National Heart, Lung &
Blood Institute

NHMRC
National Health and
Medical Research Council

NHS
National Health Service
(British)
normal horse serum
normal human serum

NHV
nursing home visit

NI
no information
not identified
not isolated

Ni
nickel

NIA
National Institute on
Aging
nephelometric inhibition
assay

NIAAA
National Institute on
Alcohol Abuse &
Alcoholism

NIAID
National Institute of
Allergy and Infectious
Diseases

NIAMSD
National Institute of
Arthritis and
Musculoskeletal and Skin
Diseases

NICHHD
National Institute of Child
Health and Human
Development

NICU
neonatal intensive care
unit

NIDA
National Institute on Drug
Abuse

NIDD
non–insulin-dependent
diabetes

NIDDKD
National Institute for Diabetes and Digestive and Kidney Diseases

NIDDM
non–insulin-dependent diabetes mellitus

NIDR
National Institute of Dental Research

NIEHS
National Institute of Environmental Health Sciences

NIF
negative inspiratory force

NIGMS
National Institute of General Medical Sciences

NIH
National Institutes of Health

NIMH
National Institute of Mental Health

NINCDS
National Institute of Neurological and Communicative Disorders and Stroke

NINDB
National Institute of Neurological Diseases and Blindness

NINR
National Institute for Nursing Research

NIOSH
National Institute of Occupational Safety and Health

NJ
nasojejunal

NK
natural killer (cells)
Nomenklatur Kommission
not known

NKA
no known allergies

NKH
nonketotic hyperosmotic

NL
normal

nl
nanoliter

NLA
neuroleptanalgesia

NLM
National Library of Medicine

NLN
National League for Nursing

NLP
neurolinguistic programming
no light perception

NLT
normal lymphocyte transfer test

NM
neuromuscular
nodular melanoma
not measurable
not measured
nuclear medicine

Nm.
L. nux moschata (nutmeg)

nm
millimicron
nanometer

NMA
National Medical
Association
neurogenic muscular
atrophy

NMI
no middle initial

NMJ
neuromuscular junction

NML
nodular mixed
histiocytic-lymphocytic
lymphoma

NMN
nicotinamide
mononucleotide

nmol
nanomole

NMP
normal menstrual period

NMR
nuclear magnetic
resonance

NMRI
Naval Medical Research
Institute

NMS
neuroleptic malignant
syndrome

NN
nurses' notes

N:N
presence of the azo group

nn.
L. nervi (nerves)

NNBA
National Nurses in
Business Association

NND
neonatal death
New and Nonofficial Drugs

NNN
Novy, MacNeal and
Nicolle's (medium)

NNS
National Natality Survey

NO
nitric oxide
none obtained

N$_2$O
dinitrogen monoxide
(nitrous oxide)

No
nobelium

No.
L. numero (to the number
of)

NOAEL
no observed adverse effect
level

Noc.
night

Noct.
L. nocte (at night)

Noct. maneq.
L. nocte maneque (at night
and in the morning)

non repetat.
L. non repetatur (do not
repeat)

NOPHN
National Organization
Public Health Nursing

NOS
not otherwise specified

NP
nasopharyngeal
nasopharynx
near point
neuropathology
neuropsychiatric
nitrogen-phosphorus

NP *(continued)*
  normal plasma
  not performed
  nucleoplasmic index
  nucleoprotein
  nurse practitioner

Np
  neptunium

NPA
  National Perinatal
    Association

NPB
  nodal premature beat

NPC
  near point of convergence
  nodal premature
    contraction
  nodal premature complex

NPCP
  National Prostatic Cancer
    Project

NPD
  Niemann-Pick disease
  nitrogen-phosphorus
    detectors
  no pathologic diagnosis

NPDB
  National Practitioner Data
    Bank

NPDL
  nodular, poorly
    differentiated
    lymphocytes
  nodular, poorly
    differentiated
    lymphocytic lymphoma

NPDR
  nonproliferative diabetic
    retinopathy

NPH
  neutral protamine
    Hagedorn (insulin)

NPH *(continued)*
  normal pressure
    hydrocephalus

NPN
  nonprotein nitrogen
  nurse's progress note

NPN compounds
  nonprotein nitrogenous
    compounds

NPO
  L. nil per os (nothing by
    mouth)

NPO/HS
  nothing by mouth at
    bedtime

4-NPP
  4-nitrophenylphosphate

NPR
  net protein ratio

Nps
  nitrophenylsulfenyl

NPT
  neoprecipitin test
  normal pressure and
    temperature

NPU
  net protein utilization

NR
  L. non repetatur (do not
    repeat)
  nonreactive
  no radiation
  no refill
  no response
  normal range
  not recorded
  not resolved

NRBC
  nucleated red blood cell

NRC
  National Research Council

NRC *(continued)*
normal retinal
correspondence
Nuclear Regulatory
Commission

NRCA
National Rehabilitation
Counseling Association

NRCC
National Registry in
Clinical Chemistry

NRD
nonrenal death

NREM
non-rapid eye movements

NREMT
National Registry of
Emergency Medical
Technicians

NRM
National Registry of
Microbiologists

nRNA
nuclear ribonucleic acid

NRS
normal rabbit serum
normal reference serum

NS
nephrotic syndrome
nerves
nervous system
neurologic survey
neurosurgery
nonspecific
nonsymptomatic
normal saline
no sample
no sequelae
not significant
not sufficient
nylon suture

N/S
normal saline

NS1
nonstructural protein 1

NS2
nonstructural protein 2

ns
nanosecond
normal saline
not significant

NSA
no serious abnormality
no significant abnormality

NSABP
National Surgical
Adjuvant Breast and
Bowel Project

NSAIA
nonsteroidal
anti-inflammatory
analgesic

NSAID
nonsteroidal
anti-inflammatory drug

NSB
nonspecific binding

NSC
no significant change
not service-connected
National Service Center

NSCD
nonservice connected
disability

NSCPT
National Society for
Cardiopulmonary
Technology

NSD
nominal single dose
nominal standard dose
(radiation)
normal spontaneous
delivery
no significant defect

NSD *(continued)*
no significant deviation
no significant difference
no significant disease

nsec
nanosecond

NSFTD
normal spontaneous
full-term delivery

NSG
nursing

nsg
nursing

NSH
National Society for
Histotechnology

NSHD
nodular sclerosing
Hodgkin's disease

NSILA
nonsuppressible
insulin-like activity

NSM
neurosecretory material

NSNA
National Student Nurse
Association

NSND
nonsymptomatic,
nondisabling

NSR
normal sinus rhythm

NSS
normal saline solution
not statistically significant

NS-ST
nonspecific ST segment

NS-ST-T
nonspecific ST segment
and T wave

NST
nonstress test

NS-T
nonspecific T wave

NSU
nonspecific urethritis

NSVD
normal spontaneous
vaginal delivery

NT
nasotracheal
neutralization test
neutralizing
nodal tachycardia
nontypable
not tested

N&T
nose and throat

nt
night

NTAB
nephrotoxic antibody

NTD
neural tube defect

NTG
nitroglycerin
nontoxic goiter

NTMI
nontransmural myocardial
infarction

NTN
nephrotoxic nephritis

NTP
5-nucleotidase
National Toxicology
Program
normal temperature and
pressure
nucleoside 5′-triphosphate

NTRS
   National Therapeutic
   Recreation Society

NTV
   nerve tissue vaccine

nU
   nanounit

Nuc
   nucleoside

NUG
   necrotizing ulcerative
   gingivitis

numc
   number concentration

numfr
   number fraction

Nur
   nitrosourea

NV
   negative variation
   neurovascular

N,V
   nausea, vomiting

N&V
   nausea and vomiting

NVA
   near visual acuity

NVD
   nausea, vomiting, and
   diarrhea
   neck vein distention
   Newcastle virus disease
   nonvalvular disease

NW
   naked weight

NWB
   non–weight-bearing

NWDL
   nodular well-differentiated
   lymphocytic lymphoma

NWTSG
   National Wilms' Tumor
   Study Group

NYD
   not yet diagnosed

nyst
   nystagmus

O

O
degree of
no
none
occiput
occlusal
office
ohne Hauch
oral
oxygen
respirations (anesthesia
chart)
vincristine (Oncovin)

O.
L. octarius (pint)
L. oculus (eye)

_O_
nonmotile organism

O_2
both eyes
diatomic (molecular)
oxygen

O_3
ozone

_o-_
ortho-

_o_
omicron

Ω
capital omega
ohm

ω
omega
angular frequency
angular velocity

OA
occipitoatlantal
occiput anterior
ocular albinism
osteoarthritis

OA *(continued)*
ovalbumin
oxalic acid

OA1
ocular albinism type 1

OA2
ocular albinism type 2

OAA
Opticians Association of
America
oxaloacetate

OAAD
ovarian ascorbic acid
depletion

OAD
obstructive airway disease

OAF
osteoclast activating factor

OAP
vincristine, cytarabine, and
prednisone
osteoarthropathy

OASDHI
Old Age, Survivors,
Disability and Health
Insurance

OAT
ornithine aminotransferase

OAV
oculoauriculovertebral
dysplasia

OAWO
opening abductory wedge
osteotomy

OB
obstetrics

O&B
opium and belladonna

OBG
    obstetrics & gynecology

OB/GYN
    obstetrics & gynecology

obl
    oblique

OBRA
    Omnibus Budget
      Reconciliation Act of
      1989

OBS
    obstetrical service
    organic brain syndrome

obs
    observed

obsd
    observed

obst
    obstetric
    obstetricians

OC
    occlusocervical
    office call
    on call
    only child
    oral contraceptive

O&C
    onset and course

Oc
    octyl

OCA
    oculocutaneous albinism

O$_2$cap
    oxygen capacity

occ
    occiput
    occipital

occup
    occupation
    occupational

OCD
    osteochondritis dissecans

OCG
    oral cholecystogram

OCP
    oral contraceptive pills

OCR
    optical character
      recognition

OCT
    ornithine
      carbamoyltransferase
    oxytocin challenge test

OD
    Doctor of Optometry
    L. oculus dexter (right eye)
    optical density
    outside diameter
    overdose

o.d.
    L. omni die (every day)

ODA
    L. occipito-dextra anterior
      (right occipito-anterior)

ODC
    orotidine 5 -phosphate
      decarboxylase

ODD
    oculodentodigital dysplasia

ODM
    ophthalmodynamometry

ODP
    L. occipito-dextra posterior
      (right occipitoposterior)

ODQ
    opponens digiti quinti

ODT
    L. occipito-dextra
      transversa (right
      occipitotransverse)

OE
on examination
otitis externa

O&E
observation and
examination

Oe
oersted

OER
oxygen enhancement ratio

OF
occipital frontal
Ovenstone factor

OFC
occipitofrontal
circumference

OFD
oral-facial-digital
(syndrome)

OG
obstetrics and gynecology

OGTT
oral glucose tolerance test

OH
hydroxyl group
outpatient

OH-Cbl
hydroxocobalamin

17-OHCS
17-hydroxycorticosteroid

OHD
organic heart disease

OHF
Omsk hemorrhagic fever

OHI
Oral Hygiene Index

OHIAA
hydroxyindoleacetic acid

OHI-S
Simplified Oral Hygiene
Index

OHP
oxygen under high
pressure

17-OHP
17-hydroxyprogesterone

OH-urea
hydroxyurea

OI
opportunistic infection
osteogenesis imperfecta

OIC
osteogenesis imperfecta
congenita

OIF
oil immersion field

OIH
orthoiodohippurate

OIHP
Office Internationale
d'Hygiene Publique

OJ
orange juice

OK
optokinetic nystagmus

OKN
opticokinetic nystagmus

OL
L. oculus laevus (left eye)
other locations

Ol.
L. oleum (oil)

OLA
L. occipito-laeva anterior
(left occipito-anterior)

OLH
ovine lactogenic hormone

Ol. oliv.
   L. oleum olivae (olive oil)

OLP
   L. occipito-laeva posterior
      (left occipitoposterior)

ol res
   oleoresin

OLT
   L. occipito-laeva transversa
      (left occipitotransverse)

OM
   obtuse marginal (coronary
      artery)
   osteomalacia
   osteomyelitis
   otitis media
   outer membrane

o.m.
   L. omni mane (every
      morning)

OMB
   Office of Management and
      Budget

OMCAA
   otitis media, catarrhal,
      acute

OMD
   ocular muscle dystrophy

OME
   otitis media with effusion

3-OMG
   3-o-methylglucose

OMI
   old myocardial infarction

OMIM
   On-Line Mendelian
      Inheritance in Man

Omn. bih.
   L. omni bihora (every two
      hours)

Omn. hor.
   L. omni hora (every hour)

Omn. noct.
   L. omni nocte (every night)

OMP
   oligo-N-methylmor-
      pholiniumpropylene
      oxide
   orotidylate
   orotidylic acid

OMPA
   octamethyl
      pyrophosphoramide
   otitis media, purulent,
      acute

OMPC
   outer membrane protein
      complex

Om. quar. hor.
   L. omni quadrante hora
      (every quarter of an hour)

OMS
   Organic mental syndrome

o.n.
   L. omni nocte (every night)

ONC
   oncology nurse, certified

ONS
   Oncology Nurses
      Association

OOB
   out of bed

OOD
   out of doors

OOLR
   ophthalmology, otology,
      laryngology, rhinology

OP
   occiput posterior
   opening pressure

OP *(continued)*
    operation
    osmotic pressure
    outpatient

O&P
    ova and parasites

op
    operation
    operative

OPC
    outpatient clinic

op cit
    L. opus citatum (in the
        work cited)

OPD
    outpatient department

o,p-DDD
    mitotane

OPG
    ocular plethysmography
    ocular pressure gradient
    oxypolygelatin

OPG/CPA
    oculoplethysmography/caro-
        tid phonoangiography

ophth
    ophthalmology

OPK
    optokinetic

OPRT
    orotate
        phosphoribosyltrans-
        ferase

OPT
    optimum
    outpatient treatment

OPV
    poliovirus vaccine live oral

OR
    operating room

ORD
    optical rotatory dispersion

Ord
    orotidine

org
    organic

ORIF
    open reduction and
        internal fixation

ORL
    otorhinolaryngology

orl
    otorhinolaryngology

Orn
    ornithine

ORO
    orotate
    orotic acid

ORT
    operating room technician

Ortho
    orthopaedics

OS
    L. oculus sinister (left eye)
    opening snap
    oral surgery

Os
    osmium

OSAS
    obstructive sleep apnea
        syndrome

OSE
    ovarian surface epithelium

Ose
    glucose

OSH
    Office on Smoking and
        Health

OSHA
> Occupational Safety and
> Health Administration

OSM
> oxygen saturation meter

OsM
> osmolar

Osm
> osmole

OT
> occlusion time
> occupational therapy
> old term
> old terminology
> old tuberculin
> original tuberculin
> orotracheal

OTC
> ornithine
> transcarbamoylase
> (ornithine
> carbamoyltrans-
> ferase)
> over the counter
> oxytetracycline

OTD
> organ tolerance dose

OTO
> otology

oto
> otology

OTR
> Ovarian Tumor Registry

OTR *(continued)*
> Registered Occupational
> Therapist

OU
> L. oculi unitas (both eyes)
> L. oculus uterque (each
> eye)

OURQ
> outer upper right quadrant

OV
> office visit

Ov
> ovary

OVD
> occlusal vertical dimension

OVLT
> organum vasculosum of the
> lamina terminalis

OW
> open wedge (osteotomy)
> out of wedlock

O/W
> oil in water
> oil-water ratio

ox
> oxymel

OXPHOS
> oxidative phosphorylation

OXT
> oxytocin

oz
> ounce

P

concentration by weight
(after optical rotations)
page
para
partial pressure
passive
paternal
peta-
pharmacopeia
phosphate group
phosphorus
plasma
poise
position
L. post (after)
posterior
postpartum
potency
premolar
presbyopia
pressure
primipara
probability
protein
pulse
punctum proximum
pupil

P.

L. post (after)

P/3

proximal third

P

Pasteurella
phosphoric residue
Plasmodium
power
pressure
probability
Proteus
radiant flux

P_1

inorganic phosphate
parental generation

P_2

pulmonic second sound

^{32}P

phosphorus 32

P_{700}

pigment in chloroplasts
bleached by light of
wavelengths about 700
nm

P_{CO_2}

carbon dioxide partial
pressure (tension)

P_i

orthophosphate

P_L

transpulmonary pressure

P_{O_2}

oxygen partial pressure
(tension)

p

page
pico-
probabilities
proton
short arm of a chromosome

p

momentum
probability
pyranose

p-

para-

p_{870}

pigment in bacterial
chromatophores bleached
by light of wavelengths
about 870 nm

$\bar{p}$

L. post (after)

π
  osmotic pressure
  the ratio of the diameter
    and circumference of a
    circle

φ
  file

Ψ
  psychiatry

ψ
  pseudouridine

PA
  paralysis agitans
  pathology
  pernicious anemia
  phakic-aphakic
  physician assistant
  posteroanterior
  prealbumin
  pregnancy-associated
  primary amenorrhea
  primary anemia
  pulmonary artery
  pulpoaxial

P&A
  percussion and
    auscultation

Pa
  pascal
  protactinium

Pa_{CO_2}
  alveolar carbon dioxide
    tension

Pa_{O_2}
  alveolar oxygen tension

Pa_{CO_2}
  arterial carbon dioxide
    tension

Pa_{O_2}
  arterial oxygen tension

PAB
  para-aminobenzoic acid

PABA
  para-aminobenzoic acid

PAC
  papular acrodermatitis of
    childhood
  political action committee
  premature atrial
    contraction
  premature auricular
    contraction
  cisplatin, doxorubicin,
    cyclophosphamide

PACIA
  particle counting
    immunoassay

PACU
  postanesthesia care unit

PAD
  preoperative autologous
    donation

P.AE.
  L. partibus aequalibus (in
    equal parts)

PAF
  paroxysmal atrial
    fibrillation
  platelet activating factor
  pulmonary arteriovenous
    fistula

PAFD
  percutaneous abscess and
    fluid drainage

PAFIB
  paroxysmal atrial
    fibrillation

PAGE
  polyacrylamide gel
    electrophoresis

PAGMK
  primary African green
    monkey kidney

PAH
    para-aminohippurate
    para-aminohippuric acid
    polycyclic aromatic
      hydrocarbon
    pulmonary artery
      hypertension

PAHA
    para-aminohippuric acid

PAHO
    Pan American Health
      Organization

PAI
    plasminogen activator
      inhibitor

PAIgG
    platelet-associated IgG

PAL
    posterior axillary line

PALA
    N-(phosphonacetyl)-L-aspart-
      ate

PALS
    pediatric advanced life
      support
    periarterial lymphoid
      sheath

PAM
    crystalline penicillin G in 2
      per cent aluminum
      monostearate
    melphalan
    phenylalanine mustard
    pralidoxime
    pulmonary alveolar
      microlithiasis
    pyridine aldoxime
      methiodide

L-PAM
    melphalan

2-PAM
    pralidoxime

Pam
    melphalan

PAN
    periodic alternating
      nystagmus
    peroxyacetyl nitrate
    polyarteritis nodosa

PANS
    puromycin
      aminonucleoside

PAO
    peak acid output

PAOD
    peripheral arterial
      occlusive disease
    peripheral arteriosclerotic
      occlusive disease

PAP
    Papanicolaou (test)
    peroxidase-antiperoxidase
    positive airway pressure
    primary atypical
      pneumonia
    prostatic acid phosphatase
    pulmonary alveolar
      proteinosis
    pulmonary artery pressure

PAPP
    p-aminopropiophenone

PAPS
    adenosine 3′-phosphate
      5′-phosphosulfate
    phosphoadenosine
      diphosphosulfate
    phosphoadenosine
      phosphosulfate
    phosphoadenosylphosphosul-
      fate

PAPVC
    partial anomalous
      pulmonary venous
      connection

PAPVR
    partial anomalous
        pulmonary venous return

PAR
    pulmonary arteriolar
        resistance

PARA
    number of pregnancies

para
    number of pregnancies

Par. aff.
    L. pars affecta (the part
        affected)

Part. aeq.
    L. partes aequales (equal
        parts)

Part. vic.
    L. partitis vicibus (in
        divided doses)

PAS
    para-aminosalicylic acid
    periodic acid-Schiff
    Professional Activity Study
    pulmonary artery stenosis

PASA
    para-aminosalicylic acid

PASB
    Pan American Sanitary
        Bureau

PAS-C
    para-aminosalicyclic acid
        crystallized with ascorbic
        acid

PASG
    pneumatic antishock
        garment

PASM
    periodic acid-silver
        methenamine

Past.
    Pasteurella

PAT
    paroxysmal atrial
        tachycardia
    pregnancy at term

pat
    patent

path.
    pathology

PAWP
    pulmonary artery wedge
        pressure

PB
    paraffin baths
    peroneus brevis
    Pharmacopoeia Britannica
        (British Pharmacopoeia)
    phenobarbital
    phonetically balanced
    pressure breathing
    protein binding
    protein-bound

P$_B$
    barometric pressure

Pb
    lead (L. plumbum)

PBA
    pulpobuccoaxial

p-bars
    parallel bars

PBC
    point of basal convergence
    primary biliary cirrhosis

PBE
    Perlsucht Bacillen
        Emulsion

PBF
    pulmonary blood flow

PBG
    pedobarograph
    porphobilinogen

PBI
 protein-bound iodine

PBL
 peripheral blood
  lymphocyte

PBN
 paralytic brachial neuritis

PBO
 penicillin in beeswax
 placebo

PBP
 penicillin-binding protein

PBPI
 penile brachial pressure
  index

PBS
 phosphate buffered saline

PBSC
 peripheral blood stem cells

PBT$_4$
 protein-bound thyroxine

PBV
 predicted blood volume
 pulmonary blood volume

PBX
 punch biopsy

PBY
 postgraduate year

PBZ
 phenylbutazone
 pyribenzamine

PC
 cisplatin and
  cyclophosphamide
 packed cells
 palmitoyl carnitine
 pentose cycle
 phosphate cycle
 phosphatidyl choline
 phosphocreatine
 platelet concentrate

PC *(continued)*
 platelet count
 portacaval
 present complaint
 printed circuit
 professional corporation
 pubococcygeus
 pulmonary capillary
 pulmonic closure

P.C.
 L. pondus civile
  (avoirdupois weight)

p.c.
 L. post cibum (after meals)

PCA
 passive cutaneous
  anaphylaxis
 patient-controlled
  analgesic
 posterior cerebral artery

PCAT
 Pharmacy college
  admission test

PCB
 paracervical block
 polychlorinated biphenyl

PcB
 near point of convergence
  to the intercentral base
  line

PCC
 pheochromocytoma
 poison control center

PCc
 periscopic concave

PCD
 phosphate-citrate-dextrose
 polycystic disease
 posterior corneal deposits

PCDD
 polychlorinated
  dibenzo-*p*-dioxins

PCDF
 polychlorinated
  dibenzofurans

PCE
 physical capacities
  evaluation

PCF
 posterior cranial fossa

PCG
 phonocardiogram

PCH
 paroxysmal cold
  hemoglobinuria

pCi
 picocurie

PCM
 protein-calorie
  malnutrition

p-**CMB**
 p-chloromercuribenzoic
  acid

PCN
 penicillin

pcn
 penicillin

PCNL
 percutaneous
  nephrostolithotomy

PCO
 polycystic ovary

PCO$_2$
 carbon dioxide production

P$_{CO_2}$
 carbon dioxide partial
  pressure (tension)

P$_{CO_2}$
 carbon dioxide partial
  pressure (tension)

pCO$_2$
 carbon dioxide partial
  pressure (tension)

p **CO$_2$**
 carbon dioxide partial
  pressure (tension)

PCP
 parachlorophenate
 pentachlorophenol
 phencyclidine
  hydrochloride
 Pneumocystis carinii
  pneumonia

PCPA
 parachlorophenylalanine

PCPQ
 Professional Corporation of
  Physicians of Quebec

PCR
 pathologically confirmed
  complete remission
 polymerase chain reaction

PCS
 portacaval shunt

pcs
 preconscious

PCT
 Patent Co-operation Treaty
 plasmacrit
 porphyria cutanea tarda
 portacaval transposition
 prothrombin consumption
  time

pct
 percent

PCTA
 percutaneous transluminal
  coronary angioplasty

PCV
 packed cell volume
 polychlorinated vinyl
 polycythemia vera

PCV-M

    myeloid metaplasia with polycythemia vera

PCVP

    procarbazine, cyclophosphamide, vinblastine, and prednisone

PCW

    pulmonary capillary wedge

PCWP

    pulmonary capillary wedge pressure

PCx

    periscopic convex

PD

    interpupillary distance
    papilla diameter
    Parkinson's disease
    patent ductus
    phosphate dehydrogenase
    plasma defect
    poorly differentiated
    postural drainage
    prism diopter
    pulmonary disease
    pulpodistal
    pupillary distance

Pd

    palladium

PDA

    Parenteral Drug Association
    patent ductus arteriosus
    posterior descending artery

PDAB

    paradimethylaminobenzalde-hyde

PDB

    Protein Data Bank

PDD

    pyridoxine-deficient diet

PDE

    paroxysmal dyspnea on exertion

PDGF

    platelet-derived growth factor

PDH

    phosphate dehydrogenase

PDI

    periodontal disease index

pDL

    predicted diffusing capacity

pdl

    pudendal

PDLL

    poorly differentiated lymphocytic lymphoma

PDP

    piperidino-pyrimidine

PDR

    Physicians' Desk Reference

PE

    paper electrophoresis
    pharyngoesophageal
    phenylephrine
    phosphatidylethanolamine
    photographic effect
    physical examination
    pleural effusion
    polyethylene
    potential energy
    pulmonary edema
    pulmonary embolism
    cisplatin, etoposide

PEBG

    phenethylbiguanide

peds

    pediatrics

PEEP
    positive end-expiratory
        pressure

PEF
    peak expiratory flow

PEFR
    peak expiratory flow rate

PEG
    pneumoencephalography
    polyethylene glycol

PEI
    phosphate excretion index
    physical efficiency index

PEL
    permissible exposure limit

Pel
    pelvis
    pelvic amputation

PEMF
    pulsating electromagnetic
        fields

pen
    penicillin

pent
    pentothal

PEO
    progressive external
        ophthalmoplegia

PEP
    phospho*enol*pyruvate
    pre-ejection period

PEPAP
    1-(2-phenethyl)-4-phenyl-4-
        acetoxypiperidine

PEPP
    positive expiratory
        pressure plateau

PER
    perineal
    protein efficiency ratio

Peritf
    peritoneal fluid

PERLA
    pupils equal, react to light
        and accommodation

Per. op. emet.
    L. peracta operatione
        emetici (when the action
        of the emetic is over)

PERRLA
    pupils equal, round,
        reactive to light and
        accommodation

PERT
    program evaluation and
        review technique

PES
    pre-excitation syndrome

PET
    polyethylene terephthalate
    positron emission
        tomography
    preeclamptic toxemia

PETE
    polyethylene terephthalate

PETG
    polyethylene terephthalate
        glycol

PETN
    pentaerythrityl
        tetranitrate

petr
    petroleum

PETT
    positron emission
        transaxial tomography

PEx
    physical examination

PF
    peritoneal fluid

PF *(continued)*
    plantar flexion
    platelet factor
    posterior fusion

pF
    picofarad

PFAS
    performic acid-Schiff
        reaction

PFC
    pelvic flexion contracture
    plaque-forming cell

PFFD
    proximal femoral focal
        deficiency

PFI
    progression-free interval

PFIB
    perfluoroisobutylene

PFK
    phosphofructokinase

PFO
    patent foramen ovale

PFR
    peak flow rate

PFT
    parafascicular
        thalamotomy
    posterior fossa tumor
    pulmonary function test

pfu
    plaque forming unit

PG
    paregoric
    Pharmacopoeia Germanica
        (German Pharmacopeia)
    phosphatidylglycerol
    plasma triglyceride
    prostaglandin
    pyoderma gangrenosum

3PG
    3-phosphoglycerate

pg
    picogram

PGA
    prostaglandin A
    pteroylglutamic acid (folic
        acid)

PGA$_1$
    prostaglandin A$_1$

PGA$_2$
    prostaglandin A$_2$

PGA$_3$
    prostaglandin A$_3$

PGB
    prostaglandin B

PGB$_1$
    prostaglandin B$_1$

PGB$_2$
    prostaglandin B$_2$

PGC
    prostaglandin C

PGC$_1$
    prostaglandin C$_1$

PGC$_2$
    prostaglandin C$_2$

PGC$_3$
    prostaglandin C$_3$

PGD
    phosphogluconate
        dehydrogenase
    phosphoglyceraldehyde
        dehydrogenase
    prostaglandin D

PGD$_1$
    prostaglandin d$_1$

PGD$_2$
    prostaglandin D$_2$
    phosphogluconate
        dehydrogenase
    plasma-glucose
        disappearance rate

PGE
prostaglandin E

PGE_1
prostaglandin E_1

PGE_2
prostaglandin E_2

PGE_3
prostaglandin E_3

PGF
prostaglandin F

PGF_1
prostaglandin F_1

$PGF_{1\alpha}$
prostaglandin F_1 alpha

PGF_2
prostaglandin F_2

$PGF_{2\alpha}$
prostaglandin F_2 alpha

PGF_3
prostaglandin F_3

PGFM
prostaglandin F and its metabolite

PGG_2
prostaglandin G_2

PGH
pituitary growth hormone
prostaglandin H

PGH_2
prostaglandin H_2

PGI
phosphoglucoisomerase
potassium, glucose, and insulin

PGI_2
prostaglandin I_2

PGK
phosphoglycerate kinase

PGM
phosphoglucomutase

pgm
picogram

PGO
ponto-geniculo-occipital

PGP
3-phosphoglyceroyl phosphate
postgamma proteinuria

PGR
psychogalvanic response

PgR
progesterone receptor

P_2Gri
diphosphoglycerate

PGTR
plasma glucose tolerance rate

PGU
postgonococcal urethritis

PH
past history
personal history
prostatic hypertrophy
public health
pulmonary hypertension

Ph
phalangeal amputation
phalanx
pharmacopeia
phenyl

Ph^1
Philadelphia chromosome

pH
acid-base scale
hydrogen ion concentration (potential of hydrogen ion)

PHA
passive hemagglutination

PHA *(continued)*
    phytohemagglutinin
    pulse height analyzer

phal
    phalanx or phalanges

phar
    pharmaceutical
    pharmacopeia
    pharmacy

Phar B
    L. Pharmaciae
    Baccalaureus (Bachelor of
    Pharmacy)

Phar C
    Pharmaceutical Chemist

Phar D
    L. Pharmaciae Doctor
    (Doctor of Pharmacy)

Phar G
    Graduate in Pharmacy

Phar M
    L. Pharmaciae Magister
    (Master of Pharmacy)

pharm
    pharmaceutical
    pharmacopeia
    pharmacy

Pharm D
    Doctor of Pharmacy

PhB
    British Pharmacopoeia

PHBB
    propylhydroxybenzyl
    benzimidazole

PhD
    Doctor of Philosophy

Phe
    phenylalanine

PhG
    Graduate in Pharmacy

PhG *(continued)*
    Pharmacopoeia Germanica
    (German Pharmacopeia)

PHI
    phosphohexoisomerase

PhI
    International
    Pharmacopoeia

PHK
    platelet
    phosphohexokinase

PHLA
    postheparin lipolytic
    activity

PhNCS
    phenylisothiocyanate

PHP
    primary
    hyperparathyroidism
    pseudohypoparathyroidism

PHPA
    p-hydroxyphenylacetate

PHPLA
    p-hydroxyphenyllactate

PHPPA
    p -hydroxyphenylpyruvic
    acid

PHPV
    persistent hyperplastic
    primary vitreous

PHS
    Public Health Service

PHx
    past history

phx
    pharynx

physiol
    physiological

PI
    parainfluenza

PI *(continued)*
    periodontal index
    phosphatidylinositol
    present illness
    protamine insulin
    pulmonary incompetence
    pulmonary infarction

pI
    point

PIA
    plasma insulin activity

PIC
    polymorphism information
    content

PICA
    posterior inferior
    cerebellar artery
    posterior inferior
    communicating artery

PICU
    pediatric intensive care
    unit
    pulmonary intensive care
    unit

PID
    pelvic inflammatory
    disease
    plasma iron disappearance
    prolapsed intervertebral
    disk

PIDT
    plasma-iron disappearance
    time

PIE
    pulmonary infiltration
    with eosinophilia
    pulmonary interstitial
    emphysema

PIF
    peak inspiratory flow
    prolactin inhibiting factor
    proliferation inhibitory
    factor

PIFR
    peak inspiratory flow rate

PIH
    prolactin-inhibiting
    hormone

PII
    plasma inorganic iodine

Pil.
    L. pilula (pill)
    L. pilulae (pills)

PIP
    phosphatidylinositol
    4-phosphate
    posterior tibial pulse
    proximal interphalangeal

PIP_2
    phosphatidylinositol
    4,5-biphosphate

PIPJ
    proximal interphalangeal
    joint

PIR
    Protein Identification
    Resource

PIT
    patellar inhibition test
    plasma iron turnover

pit
    pitocin

PITC
    phenylisothiocyanate

PITR
    plasma iron turnover rate

PIV
    parainfluenza virus

PJS
    Peutz-Jeghers syndrome

PK
    Prausnitz-Küstner
    (reaction)

PK *(continued)*
   psychokinesis
   pyruvate kinase

PKU
   phenylketonuria

PKV
   killed poliomyelitis vaccine

pkV
   peak kilovoltage

PL
   perception of light
   peroneus longus
   phospholipid
   placebo
   placental lactogen
   pulpolingual

pl
   platelets
   pleural

PLA
   pulpolinguoaxial
   pulpolabial

platinum/Vp-16
   cisplatin and etoposide

plats
   platelets

PLD
   platelet defect

PLED
   periodic lateralized
      epileptiform discharge

Pleur Fl
   pleural fluid

PLEVA
   pityriasis lichenoides et
      varioliformis acuta

PLF
   posterolateral fusion

Plf
   pleural fluid

PLIF
   posterolateral interbody
      fusion

PLP
   pyridoxal-5-phosphate

PLS
   prostaglandin-like
      substance

PLT
   primed lymphocyte typing
   psittacosis-lymphogranu-
      loma venereum-trachoma

Plt
   platelet (thrombocyte)

PLV
   live poliomyelitis vaccine
   panleukopenia virus
   phenylalanine-lysine-vaso-
      pressin
   posterior left ventricle

PM
   pacemaker
   perceptual motor
   petit mal
   photomultiplier tube
   physical medicine
   polymorph
   polymyositis
   post-mortem
   presystolic murmur
   prostate massage
   pulpomesial

Pm
   promethium

pm
   picometer

p.m.
   L. post meridiem
      (afternoon)

PMA
   papillary, marginal,
      attached

PMA *(continued)*
    paramethoxyamphetamine
    Pharmaceutical
        Manufacturers
        Association
    progressive muscular
        atrophy

PMB
    para-hydroxymercuri-
        benzoate
    polymorphonuclear
        basophil leukocytes
    postmenopausal bleeding

PMC
    pseudomembranous colitis

PMD
    personal medical doctor
    primary myocardial
        disease
    progressive muscular
        dystrophy

PME
    polymorphonuclear
        eosinophil leukocytes

PMEA
    9-(2-phosphonylmethoxy-
        ethyl)adenine

PMEDAP
    9-(2-phosphonylmethoxyeth-
        yl)-2,6-diaminopurine

PMF
    progressive massive
        fibrosis
    cisplatin, mitomycin C,
        fluorouracil

PMH
    past medical history

PMHx
    past medical history

PMI
    point of maximal impulse
    point of maximal intensity

PMI *(continued)*
    polymorphonuclear
        leukocytes
    posterior myocardial
        infarction
    progressive multifocal
        leukoencephalopathy

PMM
    pentamethylmelamine

PMMA
    polymethyl methacrylate

PMN
    polymorphonuclear
        neutrophil leukocytes

PMP
    previous menstrual period

PMR
    perinatal mortality rate
    proportionate morbidity
        ratio
    proportionate mortality
        ratio

PM&R
    physical medicine and
        rehabilitation

PMS
    phenazine methosulfate
    postmenopausal syndrome
    postmenstrual stress
    postmitochondrial
        supernatant
    pregnant mare serum
    premenstrual syndrome

PMSG
    pregnant mare serum
        gonadotropin

PMT
    point of maximum
        tenderness
    Porteus maze test
    premenstrual tension

PMW
    pokeweed mitogen

PN
- percussion note
- periarteritis nodosa
- peripheral nerve
- peripheral neuropathy
- pneumonia
- polyneuritis
- positional nystagmus
- postnatal
- progress note
- pyelonephritis

P&N
- psychiatry and neurology

Pn
- pneumonia

pn
- pneumonia

PNA
- Paris Nomina Anatomica

P_{NA}
- plasma sodium

PNC
- penicillin

PND
- paroxysmal nocturnal dyspnea
- postnasal drip

PNET
- peripheral neuroectodermal tumor

PNF
- proprioceptive neuromuscular facilitation

PNH
- paroxysmal nocturnal hemoglobinuria

PNP
- para-nitrophenol
- Pediatric Nurse Practitioner
- psychogenic nocturnal polydipsia

PNPB
- positive-negative pressure breathing

PNPP
- para-nitrophenylphosphate

PNS
- peripheral nervous system

PNU
- protein nitrogen unit

PNVX
- pneumococcus vaccine

Pnx
- pneumothorax

PO
- parieto-occipital
- L. per os (by mouth, orally)
- posterior
- postoperative

Po
- polonium

PO_4
- phosphorus (inorganic)

P_{O_2}
- oxygen partial pressure (tension)

Po_2
- oxygen partial pressure (tension)

pO_2
- oxygen partial pressure (tension)

POA
- pancreatic oncofetal antigen

POB
- phenoxybenzamine
- place of birth

POC
- postoperative care

Pocill.
      L. pocillum (a small cup)

Pocul.
      L. poculum (cup)

POD
      postoperative day

POEMS
      polyneuropathy,
        organomegaly,
        endocrinopathy,
        monoclonal gammopathy,
        and skin changes

POG
      Pediatric Oncology Group

pOH
      hydroxide ion
        concentration (potential
        of hydroxide ion)

POIK
      poikilocytosis

poik
      poikilocytosis

polio
      poliomyelitis

POLY
      polymorphonuclear
        leukocyte

poly
      polymorphonuclear
        leukocyte

poly A
      polyadenylate
      polyadenylic acid

POMP
      6-mercaptopurine,
        vincristine, methotrexate,
        and prednisone

POMR
      problem-oriented medical
        record

POMS
      Profile of Mood States

Pond.
      L. pondere (by weight)

POP
      plasma oncotic pressure
      plaster of Paris
      popliteal

POPOP
      1,4-bis(5-phenyloxazol-2-yl)
        benzene

POR
      problem-oriented record

pos
      positive

pos pr
      positive pressure

poss
      possible

post
      post mortem
      posterior

post op
      postoperative

post sag D
      posterior sagittal diameter

Post sing. sed. liq.
      L. post singulas sedes
        liquidas (after every loose
        stool)

POT
      potion

pot AGT
      potential abnormality of
        glucose tolerance

POU
      placenta, ovary, uterus

PP
      pancreatic polypeptide

PP *(continued)*
    partial pressure
    pellagra preventive
    permanent partial
    pink puffers (emphysema)
    posterior pituitary
    postpartum
    postprandial
    prothrombin-proconvertin
    protoporphyrin
    proximal phalanx
    pulse pressure
    L. punctum proximum
      (near point of
      accommodation)

PP$_i$
    pyrophosphate

P-5'-P
    pyridoxal-5-phosphate

pp
    pages

p.p.
    L. post prandium (after
      meals)

PPA
    palpation, percussion and
      auscultation
    phenylpropanolamine
    phenylpyruvic acid
    L. phiala prius agitata
      (shake well)

PPB
    parts per billion
    platelet-poor blood
    positive pressure breathing

ppb
    parts per billion

PPBS
    postprandial blood sugar

PPC
    progressive patient care

PPCA
    proserum prothrombin
      conversion accelerator

PPCF
    plasmin prothrombin
      converting factor

PPD
    paraphenylenediamine
    phenyldiphenyloxadiazole
    purified protein derivative
      (tuberculin)

ppd
    packs per day

PPD-S
    purified protein derivative,
      standard

PPF
    plasma protein fraction

ppg
    picopicogram

PPH
    postpartum hemorrhage
    primary pulmonary
      hypertension
    protocollagen proline
      hydroxylase

PPHP
    pseudopseudohypoparathyro-
      idism

PPLO
    pleuropneumonia-like
      organisms

PPM
    permanent pacemaker

ppm
    parts per million

PPNG
    penicillinase-producing
      Neisseria gonorrhoeae

PPO
    2,5-diphenyloxazole
    preferred provider
      organization

PPP

> pentose phosphate
> pathway
> platelet-poor plasma

PPPPPP

> pain, pallor, paresthesia,
> pulselessness, paralysis,
> and prostration

PPR

> Price precipitation reaction

PPRC

> Physician Payment Review
> Commission

PPRibp

> 5-phospho-α-D-ribosyl
> pyrophosphate

PPRP

> 5-phospho-α-D-ribosyl
> pyrophosphate

PPS

> pepsin
> postpartum sterilization
> postpump syndrome
> primary physician services

PPT

> plant protease test

Ppt

> precipitate
> prepared

PPTL

> postpartum tubal ligation

PPV

> positive-pressure
> ventilation

PQ

> permeability quotient
> plastoquinone
> pronator quadratus
> pyrimethamine-quinine

PQ-9

> plastoquinone-9

PR

> partial remission
> partial response
> pathology report
> pelvic rock
> peripheral resistance
> per rectum
> progesterone receptor
> progressive resistance
> prosthion
> protein
> pulse rate
> L. punctum remotum (far
> point of accommodation)

Pr

> praseodymium
> presbyopia
> prism
> propyl

PRA

> panel reactive antibodies
> plasma renin activity

P. rat. aetat.

> L. pro ratione aetatis (in
> proportion to age)

PRBC

> packed red blood cells

PRBV

> placental residual blood
> volume

PRC

> packed red cells

PRCA

> pure red cell agenesis
> pure red cell aplasia

PRD

> partial reaction of
> degeneration
> postradiation dysplasia

PRE

> progressive resistive
> exercise

PRED
  prednisone

pred
  prednisone

preg
  pregnant

pregn
  pregnancy

preop
  preoperative (before
    surgery)

prep
  preparation
  prepare (for surgery)

prepn
  preparation

PRERLA
  pupils round, equal, react
    to light and
    accommodation

pres
  president

press
  pressure

prev AGT
  previous abnormality of
    glucose tolerance

PRF
  prolactin releasing factor

PRFM
  prolonged rupture of fetal
    membranes

PRH
  prolactin-releasing
    hormone

PRI
  phosphoribose isomerase

primip
  primipara

PRL
  prolactin

Prl
  prolactin

PRM
  phosphoribomutase
  premature rupture of
    membranes
  preventive medicine

PRN
  as necessary

p.r.n.
  L. pro re nata (according as
    circumstances may
    require)

PRNT
  plaque reduction
    neutralization test

PRO
  professional review
    organization

Pro
  proline
  prothrombin

PROC
  procarbazine

Proc
  procarbazine

Proc AACR
  *Proceedings of the
    American Association for
    Cancer Research*

Proc ASCO
  *Proceedings of the
    American Society of
    Clinical Oncology*

prof
  professor
  professorship

prog
    prognosis

progn
    passive range of motion
    premature rupture of
        membranes
    prognosis
    prolonged rupture of
        membranes

ProMACE
    prednisone, methotrexate,
        doxorubicin,
        cyclophosphamide,
        etoposide

ProMACE-CytaBOM
    prednisone, methotrexate,
        doxorubicin,
        cyclophosphamide,
        etoposide, cytarabine,
        bleomycin, vincristine,
        methotrexate

ProMACE-MOPP
    prednisone, methotrexate,
        doxorubicin,
        cyclophosphamide,
        etoposide,
        mechlorethamine,
        vincristine, procarbazine,
        prednisone

ProPAC
    Prospective Payment
        Assessment Commission

Prot
    protein

pro time
    prothrombin time

pro-UK
    prourokinase

prox
    proximal

proximal/3
    proximal third

PRP
    phosphosylribitol
        phosphate
    pityriasis rubra pilaris
    platelet-rich plasma

PRPP
    phosphoribosylpyrophos-
        phate

PRRE
    pupils round, regular and
        equal

PRT
    phosphoribosyltransferase

PRTA
    proximal renal tubular
        acidosis

PRU
    peripheral resistance unit

PRV
    pseudorabies virus

PS
    pathological stage
    periodic syndrome
    phosphatidylserine
    plastic surgery
    population sample
    Porter-Silber (chromogen)
    postanesthesia shivering
    prescription
    pulmonary stenosis
    pyloric stenosis

P&S
    paracentesis and suction

P/S
    polyunsaturated-to-satu-
        rated fatty acids ratio

PS1
    polystyrene

Ps
    Pseudomonas

ps
    per second
    picosecond

PSA
    polyethylene sulfonic acid
    prostate-specific antigen
    public service
      announcement

PSC
    Porter-Silber chromogen
    posterior subcapsular
      cataract

PSCT
    peripheral stem cell
      transplantation

PSD
    peptone-starch-dextrose

PSE
    portal systemic
      encephalopathy

PSG
    peak systolic gradient
    polysomnogram
    presystolic gallop

PSGN
    poststreptococcal
      glomerulonephritis

psi
    pounds per square inch

PSIS
    posterosuperior iliac spine

PSL
    parasternal line

PSM
    presystolic murmur

PSMF
    protein sparing modified
      fast

PSP
    periodic short pulse
    phenolsulfonphthalein

PSP *(continued)*
    positive spike pattern
    progressive supranuclear
      palsy

PSRO
    Professional Standards
    Review Organization

PSS
    physiologic saline solution
    progressive systemic
      sclerosis

PST
    penicillin, streptomycin
      and tetracycline

PSU
    primary site undetermined

PSV
    pressure support
      ventilation

PSVT
    paroxysmal
      supraventricular
      tachycardia

PSW
    psychiatric social worker

PT
    parathyroid
    paroxysmal tachycardia
    patient
    phototoxicity
    physical therapist
    physical therapy
    pneumothorax
    posterior tibial
    pronator teres
    prothrombin time

Pt
    patient
    platinum

pt
    pint
    point

PTA
    percutaneous transluminal
        angioplasty
    persistent truncus
        arteriosus
    phosphotungstic acid
    plasma thromboplastin
        antecedent (blood
        coagulation Factor XI)
    posttraumatic amnesia
    posttraumatic arthritis
    prior to admission

PTAH
    phosphotungstic acid
        hematoxylin

PTB
    patellar tendon bearing
    prior to birth

PTC
    percutaneous transhepatic
        cholangiogram
    percutaneous transhepatic
        cholangiography
    phenylthiocarbamide
    phenylthiocarbamoyl
    plasma thromboplastin
        component (blood
        coagulation Factor IX)

PTCA
    percutaneous transluminal
        coronary angioplasty

PTD
    permanent and total
        disability

Ptd
    phosphatidyl

PtdCho
    phosphatidylcholine

PtdEth
    phosphatidylethanolamine

PtdIns
    phosphatidylinositol

PtdSer
    phosphatidylserine

PTE
    parathyroid extract
    pulmonary
        thromboembolism

PTED
    pulmonary
        thromboembolic disease

PTEN
    pentaerythritol
        tetranitrate

PTF
    plasma thromboplastin
        factor

PTFE
    polytetrafluoroethylene

PTH
    parathormone
    parathyroid hormone
    post-transfusion hepatitis

PTHS
    parathyroid hormone
        secretion (rate)

PTI
    persistent tolerant
        infection

PTM
    post-transfusion
        mononucleosis

PTMA
    phenyltrimethylammonium

PTO
    Perlsucht Tuberculin
        original

PTP
    post-tetanic potentiation
    posttransfusion purpura

PTR
    peripheral total resistance

PTR *(continued)*
Perlsucht Tuberculin Rest

PTS
para-toluenesulfonic acid

PTSD
posttraumatic stress
disorder

PTSM
pyruvaldehyde-bis-(*N*-4-
methylthiosemicarbazone)-

PTT
activated partial
thromboplastin time
partial thromboplastin
time
particle transport time
patellar tendon transfer

PTU
propylthiouracil

PTX
parathyroidectomy

PTZ
pentylenetetrazol

PU
peptic ulcer
pregnancy urine

Pu
plutonium

PUBS
percutaneous umbilical
cord blood sampling

PUD
peptic ulcer disease
pulmonary disease

PUE
pyrexia of unknown
etiology

PUFA
polyunsaturated fatty acid

pul
pulmonary

PULM
L. pulmentum (gruel)

pulm
pulmonary

pulv.
L. pulvis (powder)

PUMC
Peking Union Medical
College

PUO
pyrexia of unknown origin

PUPPP
pruritic urticarial papules
and plaques of pregnancy

Pur
purine

PUVA
psoralen plus ultraviolet A

PV
peripheral vascular
peripheral vein
peripheral vessels
plasma volume
polycythemia vera
portal vein
postvoiding

P&V
pyloroplasty and vagotomy

p.v.
per vaginam (through the
vagina)

PVA
polyvinyl alcohol

PVB
cisplatin, vinblastine,
bleomycin

PVC
polyvinyl chloride
postvoiding cystogram
premature ventricular
contraction

PVC *(continued)*
    pulmonary venous
        congestion

PVD
    peripheral vascular disease

PVE
    prosthetic valve
        endocarditis

PVF
    portal venous flow

PVM
    pneumonia virus of mice

PVO
    pyogenic vertebral
        osteomyelitis

PVP
    penicillin V potassium
    peripheral vein plasma
    polyvinylpyrrolidone
    portal venous pressure

PVP-I
    povidone-iodine

PVR
    peripheral vascular
        resistance
    pulmonary vascular
        resistance

PVS
    premature ventricular
        systole

PVT
    paroxysmal ventricular
        tachycardia
    portal vein thrombosis

pvt
    private

PW
    plantar wart

PW *(continued)*
    posterior wall

PWA
    person with AIDS

PWB
    partial weight bearing

PWI
    posterior wall infarct

PWM
    pokeweed mitogen

PWP
    pulmonary wedge pressure

PX
    physical examination

px
    physical examination
    pneumothorax

PXE
    pseudoxanthoma elasticum

Pxl
    pyridoxal

Pxm
    pyridoxamine

PYLL
    potential years of life lost

Pyr
    pyrimidine

PZ
    pancreozymin

PZA
    pyrazinamide

PZ-CCK
    pancreozymincholecysto-
        kinin

PZI
    protamine zinc insulin

Q

Q

coenzyme Q
coulomb
quantity
ubiquinone

Q

electric charge
heat
quantity
reaction quotient

Q_{10}

temperature coefficient
ubiquinone

Q_B

total body clearance

$\dot{Q}$

rate of blood flow

q

long arm of a chromosome

q.

L. quaque (each, every)

q

electric charge
probability of an
    alternative event
quantity
ubiquinone

QA

quality assurance

q.a.

quality assurance

QAM

every morning

QC

quality control
quinine-colchicine

Q_{CO_2}

the microliters STPD of
    CO_2 given off per
    milligram of tissue per
    hour

q.d.

L. quaque die (every day)

q 28 days

every 28 days

q.d.s.

L. quater die sumendum
    (to be taken four times a
    day)

$Q\text{-}H_2$

ubiquinol

q.h.

L. quaque hora (every
    hour)

q2h

L. quaque secunda hora
    (every two hours)

q4h

L. quaque quarta hora
    (every four hours)

q.h.s.

L. quaque hora somni
    (every bedtime)

q.i.d.

L. quater in die (four times
    a day)

QJM

Quarterly Journal of
    Medicine

q.l.

L. quantum libet (as much
    as desired)

q.m.

L. quaque mane (every
    morning)

q month
    each month

QMT
    quantitative muscle testing

q.n.
    L. quaque nocte (every
        night)

QNS
    quantity not sufficient
    Queen's Nursing Sister (of
        Queen's Institute of
        District Nursing)

qns
    quantity not sufficient

Q_O
    oxygen consumption

QO_2
    oxygen quotient

Q_{O_2}
    oxygen consumption

q.o.d.
    every other day

QP
    quanti-Pirquet (reaction)

q.p.
    L. quantum placeat (as
        much as desired)

q.p.m.
    every afternoon or evening

q.q.h.
    L. quaque quarta hora
        (every four hours)

Qq.hor.
    L. quaque hora (every
        hour)

qqv
    L. quae vide (which see,
        plural)

QRS
    Q wave, R wave, and S
        wave

QRZ
    wheal reaction time

QS_2
    electromechanical systole

q.s.
    L. quantum satis (sufficient
        quantity)

q.suff.
    L. quantum sufficit (as
        much as suffices)

qt.
    quart

quad
    quadriceps
    quadrilateral
    quadriplegic

quad atrophy
    quadriceps atrophy

quadrupl.
    L. quadruplicato (four
        times as much)

quant
    quantity

Quat.
    L. quattuor (four)

quat.
    L. quattuor (four)

QUICHA
    quantitative inhalation
        challenge apparatus

Quinq.
    L. quinque (five)

Quint.
    L. quintus (fifth)

Quotid.
    L. quotidie (daily)

q 4 wk
    every 4 weeks

q.v.
    L. quantum vis (as much as
    you please)

q.v. *(continued)*
    L. quod vide (which see)

R
  Behnken's unit
  radical
  radius, complete
    (congenital absence of
    limb)
  Rankine scale
  rate
  Réaumur scale
  rectal
  regression coefficient
  resistance
  respiration
  respiratory exchange ratio
  rhythm
  right
  Rinne test
  roentgen
  rough (colony)
  rub

R.
  L. remotum (far)

R
  gas constant
  resistance
  Rickettsia

℞
  L. recipe (take)
  prescription
  therapy
  treatment

R$_A$
  airway resistance

R$_{AW}$
  airway resistance

R$_e$
  Reynold's number

R$_f$
  symbol denoting movement
    of a substance in paper
    chromatography relative
    to the solvent front

R$_s$
  resolution

R✓
  receipt done

r
  drug resistance
  radius, incomplete
    (congenital absence of
    limb)
  recombinant
  ring chromosome
  applied shear stress

r
  correlation coefficient
  distance radius
  drug resistance

r$_s$
  Spearman's rank
    correlation coefficient

r-
  racemic

ρ
  correlation coefficient
  electric charge density
  mass density

RA
  radium
  regular army
  renal artery
  repeat action
  rheumatoid arthritis
  right anterior
  right arm
  right atrium
  right auricle

Ra
  radium

RAAGG
  rheumatoid arthritis
    agglutination

RAD
   reactive airway disease
   right axis deviation

rad
   absorbed dose of ionizing
      radiation
   radial
   radian

rad.
   L. radix (root)

RADTS
   rabbit antidog thymus
      serum

RAE
   right atrial enlargement

RAF
   rheumatoid arthritis factor

RAH
   regressing atypical
      histiocytosis
   right atrial hypertrophy

RAI
   radioactive iodine

RAIU
   radioactive iodine uptake

RAM
   random access memory
   random alternating
      movements

RAMC
   Royal Army Medical Corps

RAMT
   rabbit antimouse
      thymocyte

RAO
   right anterior oblique

RAP
   right atrial pressure

RAPS
   Rapid Acute Physiology
      Score

RARLS
   rabbit antirat lymphocyte
      serum

RAS
   renal artery stenosis
   reticular activating system

RA slide
   rheumatoid arthritis slide
      test

RAST
   radioallergosorbent test

RATG
   rabbit antithymocyte
      globulin

RATHAS
   rat thymus antiserum

RATx
   radiation therapy

RAV
   Rous-associated virus

RAW
   airway resistance

RB
   respiratory bronchiole

Rb
   rubidium

RBA
   rose bengal antigen

RBB
   retrobulbar block
   right bundle branch

RBBB
   right bundle branch block

RBC
   red blood cell
   red blood (cell) count

RBC/hpf
   red blood cells per high
      power field

RBC IT
red blood cell iron turnover

RBCM
red blood cell mass

RBCV
red blood cell volume

RBD
right border of dullness

RBE
relative biological
effectiveness

RBF
renal blood flow

RBL
Reid's base line

RBP
retinol binding protein

RBRVS
resource-based relative
value scale

RBS
random blood sugar

Rbu
ribulose

Rby
ribitol

RC
red cell
red cell casts
retrograde cystogram

RCA
right coronary artery

RCBV
regional cerebral blood
volume

RCC
red cell count

RCD
relative cardiac dullness

RCF
red cell folate
relative centrifugal force

RCM
red cell mass
right costal margin
Royal College of Midwives

RCN
Royal College of Nursing

RCO
aliphatic acyl radical

RCOG
Royal College of
Obstetricians and
Gynaecologists

RCP
Royal College of Physicians

rcp
reciprocal translocation

RCP(E) or (Edin)
Royal College of Physicians
(Edinburgh)

RCP(I)
Royal College of Physicians
(Ireland)

RCPSC
Royal College of Physicians
and Surgeons of Canada

RCR
respiratory control ratio

RCS
reticulum cell sarcoma
Royal College of Surgeons

RCS(E) or (Edin)
Royal College of Surgeons
(Edinburgh)

RCS(I)
Royal College of Surgeons
(Ireland)

RCU
red cell utilization

RCV
red cell volume

RCVS
Royal College of
Veterinary Surgeons

RD
Raynaud's disease
reaction of degeneration
resistance determinant
respiratory disease
retinal detachment
right deltoid
right dorsoanterior

rd
rutherford

RDA
recommended daily
allowance
recommended dietary
allowance
right dorsoanterior
position of the fetus

RDE
receptor destroying
enzyme

RDFS
ratio of decayed and filled
surfaces

RDH
Registered Dental
Hygienist

RDI
rupture-delivery interval

RDP
right dorsoposterior
position of the fetus

RDS
respiratory distress
syndrome
respiratory distress
syndrome of the newborn

RDW
red cell distribution width

RE
radium emanation
random error
rectal examination
regional enteritis
reticuloendothelial
retinol equivalent
right eye

Re
rhenium

REA
radioenzymatic assay

REC
record
recreation

rec
record
recreation

recip
recipient

recryst
recrystallize

RECT
rectum

Rect.
L. rectificatus (rectified)

rect
rectum

Redig. in pulv.
L. redigatur in pulverem
(let it be reduced to
powder)

Red. in pulv.
L. reductus in pulverem
(reduced to powder)

REE
resting energy expenditure

REF
　　renal erythropoietic factor

ref
　　reference

REG
　　radioencephalogram

REG UMB
　　umbilical region

rehab
　　rehabilitation

REL
　　recommended exposure
　　　limit

rel
　　relative

REM
　　rapid eye movements

rem
　　roentgen equivalent man

REMP
　　roentgen-equivalent-man
　　　period

ren
　　renal

ren∠
　　renal angle

Rep.
　　L. repetatur (let it be
　　　repeated)

rep
　　report
　　roentgen equivalent
　　　physical

RER
　　renal excretion rate
　　rough endoplasmic
　　　reticulum

RES
　　resident
　　reticuloendothelial system

res
　　research
　　resident

Resp
　　respiratory rate

resp
　　respectively
　　respiration
　　respiratory

retic
　　reticulocyte

REV
　　reticuloendotheliosis
　　　viruses

RF
　　Reitland-Franklin (unit)
　　relative fluorescence
　　releasing factor
　　rheumatic fever
　　rheumatoid factor

RFA
　　right femoral artery
　　right forearm
　　right frontoanterior

RFB
　　retained foreign body

RFL
　　right frontolateral

RFLA
　　rheumatoid factor–like
　　　activity

RFLP
　　restriction fragment length
　　　polymorphism

RFP
　　right frontoposterior

RFPS(Glasgow)
  Royal Faculty of
    Physicians and Surgeons
    of Glasgow

RFS
  relapse-free survival
  renal function study

RFT
  right frontotransverse

RFW
  in cardiology, rapid filling
    wave

RG
  right gluteal

RGN
  Registered General Nurse
    (Scotland)

RH
  reactive hyperemia
  relative humidity
  releasing hormone
  right hand
  right hyperphoria

Rh
  rhesus factor
  rheumatoid
  rheumatology
  rhodium

rh
  rheumatic

RHBF
  reactive hyperemia blood
    flow

RHD
  relative hepatic dullness
  rheumatic heart disease

rheum.
  rheumatic
  rheumatism
  rheumatoid

RHF
  right heart failure

RHL
  right hepatic lobe

RHLN
  right hilar lymph node

rhm
  roentgen (per) hour (at one)
    meter

Rh neg
  Rhesus factor negative

Rh pos
  Rhesus factor positive

RHS
  right hand side

r-HuEPO
  recombinant human
    erythropoietin

RI
  recession index
  refractive index
  regional ileitis
  respiratory illness

RIA
  radioimmunoassay

Rib
  ribose

RIC
  Royal Institute of
    Chemistry

RICM
  right intercostal margin

RICU
  respiratory intensive care
    unit

RID
  radial immunodiffusion

RIF
  right iliac fossa

RIFA
  radioiodinated fatty acid

RIH
right inguinal hernia

RIHSA
radioactive iodine–tagged
human serum albumin

RIPHH
Royal Institute of Public
Health and Hygiene

RIR
right iliac region

RISA
radioactive iodinated
serum albumin

RIST
radioimmunosorbent test

RITC
rhodamine isothiocyanate

RIU
radioactive iodine uptake

RK
rabbit kidney
right kidney

RKY
roentgenkymography

RL
right leg
right lung
Ringer's lactate

R⁻L
right to left

RLBCD
right lower border of
cardiac dullness

RLC
Rapoport-Luebering cycle
residual lung capacity

RLD
related living donor

RLE
right lower extremity

RLF
retrolental fibroplasia

RLL
radiolucent line
right lower limb
right lower lobe

RLN
recurrent laryngeal nerve

RLP
radiation-leukemia-
protection

RLQ
right lower quadrant

RLS
Ringer's lactate solution

RM
radical mastectomy
reference material
repetition maximum
respiratory movement

R&M
routine and microscopic

RMA
right mentoanterior

RMCA
right middle cerebral
artery

RMK
rhesus monkey kidney

RML
right middle lobe

RMP
rapidly miscible pool
resting membrane
potential
right mentoposterior

RMS
root-mean-square
Ruvalcaba-Myrhe-Smith
(syndrome)

RMSF
　　Rocky Mountain spotted
　　fever

RMT
　　retromolar trigone
　　right mentotransverse

RMV
　　respiratory minute volume

RN
　　Registered Nurse

Rn
　　radon

RNA
　　radionuclide angiography
　　ribonucleic acid

RNase
　　ribonuclease

RNC
　　registered nurse clinician

RND
　　radical neck dissection

RNP
　　registered nurse
　　practitioner
　　ribonucleoprotein

RO
　　Ritter-Oleson (technique)
　　routine order

R/O
　　rule out

ROA
　　right occipitoanterior

ROC
　　receiver operating
　　characteristics

ROD
　　renal osteodystrophy

ROH
　　rat ovarian hyperemia
　　(test)

ROI
　　region of interest
　　right occipitolateral

ROM
　　range of motion
　　read-only memory
　　right otitis media
　　rupture of membranes

ROP
　　right occipitoposterior

ROS
　　review of systems

ROT
　　remedial occupational
　　therapy
　　right occipitotransverse

RP
　　(certificate in) radiological
　　physics
　　radial pulse
　　reactive protein
　　refractory period
　　resting pressure
　　retrograde pyelogram

Rp
　　pulmonary resistance

RPA
　　right pulmonary artery

RPCF
　　Reiter protein complement
　　fixation

RPCFT
　　Reiter protein
　　complement-fixation test

RPCH
　　rural primary care hospital

RPE
　　retinal pigment epithelium

RPF
　　relaxed pelvic floor
　　renal plasma flow

RPG
retrograde pyelogram

RPGN
rapidly progressive
glomerulonephritis

R Ph
Registered Pharmacist

RPI
reticulocytic production
index

rpm
revolutions per minute

RPMI
Roswell Park Memorial
Institute

RPN
resident's progress note

RPO
right posterior oblique

RPP
rate-pressure product

RPR
rapid plasma reagin (test)

RPRC
rapid plasma reagin card
test

RPS
renal pressor substance

RPV
right pulmonary veins

RQ
recovery quotient
respiratory quotient

RR
radiation response
rate-responsive (pacemaker
code)
recovery room
relative risk
renin release
respiratory rate

RR *(continued)*
response rate

R&R
rate and rhythm
rest and recuperation

RRA
radioreceptor assay
Registered Record
Administrator

RRE
round, regular, and equal

RR&E
round, regular, and equal

RR-HPO
rapid recompression—high
pressure oxygen

RRL
Registered Record
Librarian

rRNA
ribosomal RNA

RRP
relative refractory period

RRR
renin-release rate

RRV
rhesus monkey rotavirus

RS
Reed-Sternberg cell
Reiter's syndrome
respiratory syncytial
(virus)
right side
Ringer's solution

RSA
relative specific activity
reticulum cell sarcoma
right sacroanterior
roentgen stereophoto-
grammetric analysis

RSB
right sternal border

RSC
rested-state contraction

RScA
right scapuloanterior

RSCN
Registered Sick Children's
Nurse

RScP
right scapuloposterior

RSD
reflex sympathetic
dystrophy
relative standard deviation

RSDV
respiratory
sialodacryoadenitis virus

RSE
reference standard
endotoxin

RSM
Royal Society of Medicine

RSNA
Radiological Society of
North America

RSP
right sacroposterior

RSR
regular sinus rhythm

RSS
Russian spring-summer
(encephalitis)

RST
radiosensitivity test
right sacrotransverse

RSTMH
Royal Society of Tropical
Medicine and Hygiene

RSV
respiratory syncytial virus
right subclavian vein
Rous sarcoma virus

RT
radiation therapy
reaction time
recreational therapy
registered technician
respiratory therapy
right
right thigh
room temperature

RT$_3$
reverse triiodothyronine

RTA
renal tubular acidosis

RTC
return to clinic

RTD
routine test dilution

RTF
replication and transfer
residential treatment
facility
resistance transfer factor
respiratory tract fluid

RT + 5-Fu
radiation therapy and
5-fluorouracil

rTMP
ribothymidylic acid

RTOG
Radiation Therapy
Oncology Group

rt-PA
recombinant tissue
plasminogen activator

RUR
resin-uptake ratio

RURTI
recurrent upper
respiratory tract infection

RU
rat unit

RU *(continued)*
    resistance unit
    retrograde ureterogram

Ru
    ruthenium

RUE
    right upper extremity

RUG
    retrograde ureterogram

RUL
    right upper limb
    right upper lobe
    right upper lung

RUOQ
    right upper outer quadrant

RUQ
    right upper quadrant

RV
    rat virus
    Rauscher virus, associated
      disease
    recreational vehicle
    residual volume
    respiratory volume
    return visit
    right ventricle
    rubella virus

RVA
    rabies vaccine, adsorbed

RVB
    red venous blood

RVD
    relative vertebral density

RVE
    right ventricular
      enlargement

RVEDP
    right ventricular
      end-diastolic pressure

RVH
    right ventricular
      hypertrophy

RVI
    relative value index

RVO
    relaxed vaginal outlet

RVR
    renal vascular resistance
    resistance to venous return

RVRA
    renal vein renin activity
    renal venous renin assay

RVRC
    renal vein renin
      concentration

RVS
    relative value scale

RVT
    renal vein thrombosis

RV/TLC
    residual volume to total
      lung capacity ratio

RVVL
    rubella virus vaccine live

RW
    ragweed

℞
    L. recipe, take

S

sacral vertebrae (S1–S5)
serum
siemens
single
smooth (colony)
soluble
sone
spherical lens
substrate
sulfur
supravergence
Svedberg unit

S.

L. signa (mark)

S

entropy
Salmonella
Schistosoma
Spirillum
standard
Staphylococcus
Streptococcus

S₁

first heart sound

S₂

second heart sound

S₂ₚ

symbol for the pulmonic
valve closure component
of the second heart sound

S₃

third heart sound
ventricular gallop

S₄

fourth heart sound
atrial gallop

Sf

Svedberg flotation unit

Ŝ

in electrocardiology,
symbol for spatial vector

s

second
single
standard deviation

s.

L. semis (half)
L. sinister (left)

s.

L. sine (without)

s

sample standard deviation
symmetrical

s⁻¹

reciprocal second

Σ

sigmoid
sigmoidoscopy

σ

standard deviation

SA

salicylic acid
sarcoma
secondary amenorrhea
secondary anemia
serum albumin
sinoatrial
sinus arrest
Stokes-Adams (disease)
surface area
sustained action

S.A.

L. secundum artem
(according to art)

S-A

salicylic acid
sinoatrial
surface area
sustained action

S/A
   sugar and acetone

S&A
   sugar and acetone

SAA
   severe aplastic anemia

SAAABB
   Subcommittee on
      Accreditation of the
      American Association of
      Blood Banks

SAB
   significant asymptomatic
      bacteriuria
   subarachnoid block

S-AB
   sinoatrial block

SAC
   short-arm cast

SACD
   subacute combined
      degeneration

SACH
   single axis cushion heel
      (foot)

SACT
   sinoatrial conduction time

SAECG
   signal-averaged
      electrocardiogram

SAF
   serum accelerator factor

SAG
   Swiss-type
      agammaglobulinemia

SAH
   S-adenoxyl homocysteine
   subarachnoid hemorrhage

SAKK
   Swiss Group for Clinical
      Cancer Research

SAL
   salicylate

S.A.L.
   L. secundum artis leges
      (according to the rules of
      art)

sal
   salicylate
   saline
   saliva

SAM
   systolic anterior motion
   sulfated acid
      mucopolysaccharide

SAN
   sinoatrial node

SANC
   short-arm navicular cast

SAO$_2$
   arterial oxygen percent
      saturation

SAP
   serum alkaline
      phosphatase
   systemic arterial pressure

sapon
   saponification

SAPS
   Simplified Acute
      Physiology Score

SART
   sinoatrial recovery time

SAS
   short-arm splint
   Statistical Analysis System
   supravalvular aortic
      stenosis

SAT
   Scholastic Aptitude Test
   saturated

sat
 saturated

SATA
 spatial average temporal
  average

sat. sol.
 saturated solution

sat. soln.
 saturated solution

SB
 serum bilirubin
 sinus bradycardia
 small bowel
 Stanford-Binet
 sternal border
 stillbirth

Sb
 antimony (L. stibium)

SbCl$_3$
 antimony trichloride

SBDCo
 single-breath diffusing
  capacity for carbon
  monoxide

SBE
 shortness of breath on
  exertion
 subacute bacterial
  endocarditis

SBF
 splanchnic blood flow

SBFT
 small bowel follow through

SBI
 serious bacterial infection

SBN
 single-breath nitrogen
  (test)

SBO
 small bowel obstruction

Sb$_2$O$_3$
 antimony trioxide

Sb$_2$O$_5$
 antimony pentoxide

Sb$_4$O$_6$
 antimony trioxide

SBOM
 soybean oil meal

SBP
 scleral buckling procedure
 systemic blood pressure
 systolic blood pressure

SBTI
 soybean trypsin inhibitor

SBW
 spectral bandwidth

SC
 closure of the semilunar
  valves
 sacrococcygeal
 secretory component
 self care
 sickle cell
 sternoclavicular
 subcutaneous
 succinylcholine

Sc
 scandium

sc
 subcutaneous
 subcutaneously

SCA
 sickle cell anemia

SCAB
 streptozotocin, lomustine,
  doxorubicin, and
  bleomycin sulfate

SCAT
 sheep cell agglutination
  test
 sickle cell anemia test

SCC
squamous cell cancer
squamous cell carcinoma

SCD
subacute combined
degeneration
sudden cardiac death
sudden coronary death

ScD
Doctor of Science

ScDA
L. scapulodextra anterior
(right scapuloanterior)

ScDP
L. scapulodextra posterior
(right scapuloposterior)

SCFE
slipped capital femoral
epiphysis

SCG
serum chemistry graft
sodium cromoglycate

SCH
sole community hospital
succinylcholine

SChE
acylcholine acylhydrolase

SCHIZ
schizophrenia

schiz
schizophrenia

SCI
spinal cord injury

sci
science

SCID
severe combined
immunodeficiency

SCIPP
sacrococcygeal to inferior
pubic point

SCJ
squamocolumnar junction

SCK
serum creatine kinase

ScLA
L. scapulolaeva anterior
(left scapuloanterior)

ScLP
L. scapulolaeva posterior
(left scapuloposterior)

SCM
Society of Computer
Medicine
State Certified Midwife
sternocleidomastoid

SCN
thiocyanate

SCOP
scopolamine

scop
scopolamine

SCP
single-celled protein

SCPK
serum creatine
phosphokinase

SCR
silicon-controlled rectifier

scr
scruple

SCS
silicon-controlled switch

SCT
sex chromatin test
staphylococcal clumping
test

SCU
special care unit

SCUBA
   self-contained underwater
      breathing apparatus

scu-PA
   single chain
      urokinase-type
      plasminogen activator

SD
   septal defect
   serologically defined
   serum defect
   shoulder disarticulation
   skin dose
   spontaneous delivery
   Sprague-Dawley (rat)
   stable disease
   standard deviation
   streptodornase
   sudden death

S/D
   systolic to diastolic

SDA
   L. sacrodextra anterior
      (right sacroanterior)
   specific dynamic action

S-D curve
   strength-duration curve

SDD
   sterile dry dressing

SDE
   specific dynamic effect

SDH
   serine dehydrase
   sorbitol dehydrogenase
   succinate dehydrogenase
   subdural hematoma

SDI
   standard deviation interval
      (index)

SDM
   standard deviation of the
      mean

SDMS
   Society of Diagnostic
      Medical Sonographers

SDP
   L. sacrodextra posterior
      (right sacroposterior)

SDR
   surgical dressing room

SDS
   Self-Rating Depression
      Scale
   sodium dodecyl sulfate
   standard deviation scores
   sudden death syndrome

SDS-PAGE
   sodium dodecyl
      sulfate–polyacrylamide
      gel electrophoresis

SDT
   L. sacrodextra transversa
      (right sacrotransverse)

SE
   saline enema
   side effects
   sphenoethmoidal suture
   standard error
   Starr-Edwards (valve)
   systematic error

Se
   selenium

sec
   second

sec
   secondary

SED
   skin erythema dose
   spondyloepiphyseal
      dysplasia

sed rate
   sedimentation rate

sed rt.
    sedimentation rate

SEE
    standard error of the
        estimate

SEG
    sonoencephalogram
    Southeastern Cancer Study
        Group

seg
    segmented (leukocyte)

SEM
    scanning electron
        microscope
    scanning electron
        microscopy
    standard error of the mean

semel in d.
    L. semel in die (once a day)

Semf
    seminal fluid

SEMI
    subendocardial myocardial
        infarction

Semih.
    L. semihora (half an hour)

SEOG
    Southeastern Oncology
        Group

SEP
    sensory evoked potential
    somatosensory evoked
        potential
    systolic ejection period

sep
    separated

sepn
    separation

Sept.
    L. septem (seven)

SEQ
    L. sequela (that which
        follows)

seq
    L. sequela (that which
        follows)
    sequestrum

seq. luce
    L. sequenti luce (the
        following day)

SER
    smooth endoplasmic
        reticulum
    somatosensory evoked
        response
    systolic ejection rate

Ser
    serine

Serv.
    L. serva (keep, preserve)

SES
    socioeconomic status

Sesquih.
    L. sesquihora (an hour and
        a half)

SET
    systolic ejection time

SF
    scarlet fever
    spinal fluid
    synovial fluid

Sf
    spinal fluid
    Svedberg flotation unit

sfc
    spinal fluid count

SFD
    skin-film distance

SFEMG
    single fiber
        electromyography

SFP
> screen filtration pressure
> spinal fluid pressure

SFS
> split function study

SFW
> slow filling wave

SG
> serum globulin
> skin graft
> specific gravity

S-G
> Sachs-Georgi (test)

SG$_{AW}$
> specific airways
> conductance

SGA
> small for gestational age
> student government
> association

SGO
> Surgeon General's Office

SGOT
> serum glutamic-oxaloacetic
> transaminase

SGP
> serine glycerophosphatide

SGPT
> serum glutamate pyruvate
> transaminase

SH
> serum hepatitis
> sex hormone
> shoulder
> sinus histiocytosis
> social history
> sulfhydryl
> surgical history

S&H
> speech and hearing

Sh
> shoulder
> shoulder amputation

SHB
> sulfhemoglobin

SHBD
> serum hydroxybutyrate
> dehydrogenase

SHBG
> sex hormone–binding
> globulin

SHG
> synthetic human gastrin

Shk
> shikimic acid

SHO
> secondary hypertrophic
> osteoarthropathy

Shy
> 6-mercaptopurine

SI
> sacroiliac
> saturation index
> self-inflicted
> seriously ill
> serum iron
> soluble insulin
> stimulation index
> stroke index
> Système International
> d'Unites (International
> System of Units)

Si
> silicon

Sia
> sialic acid

SIADH
> syndrome of inappropriate
> antidiuretic hormone

SICD
> serum isocitric
> dehydrogenase

SID
    sudden infant death

s.i.d.
    L. semel in die (once a day)

SIDS
    sudden infant death
        syndrome

SIg
    surface immunoglobulin

Sig.
    L. signetur (let it be
        labeled)

Sig. n. pro.
    L. signa nomine proprio
        (label with the proper
        name)

SIJ
    sacroiliac joint

SIM
    selected ion monitoring

simul
    at the same time

SIMV
    synchronized intermittent
        mandatory ventilation

sing.
    L. singulorum (of each)

Si non val.
    L. si non valeat (if it is not
        enough)

Si op. sit
    L. si opus sit (if it is
        necessary)

SIP
    Sickness Impact Profile

SIRS
    soluble immune response
        suppressor

SISI
    short increment sensitivity
        index

Si vir. perm.
    L. si vires permittant (if
        the strength will permit)

SIW
    self-inflicted wound

SJR
    Shinowara-Jones-Reinhard
        (unit)

SK
    streptokinase

SKSD
    streptokinase-streptodor-
        nase

SL
    sensation level
    serious list
    Sibley-Lehninger (unit)
    slight
    streptolysin
    sublingual

sL
    sublingual

sl
    sublingual
    slight
    slyke

SLA
    L. sacrolaeva anterior (left
        sacroanterior)
    slide latex agglutination
    swine lymphocyte antigens

SLB
    short-leg brace

SLC
    short-leg cast

SLD
    serum lactic
        dehydrogenase

SLDH

serum lactic
dehydrogenase

SLE

St. Louis encephalitis
systemic lupus
erythematosus

SLEV

St. Louis encephalitis virus

SLI

splenic localization index

SLKC

superior limbic
keratoconjunctivitis

SLN

superior laryngeal nerve

SLO

streptolysin-O

SLP

L. sacrolaeva posterior (left
sacroposterior)

SLR

straight leg raising
Streptococcus lactis R

SLRT

straight leg raising test

SLS

segment long-spacing
(collagen)
short-leg splint

SLT

L. sacrolaeva transversa
(left sacrotransverse)

SM

streptomycin
submucous
suction method
systolic mean
systolic murmur

Sm

samarium

SMA

Sequential Multiple
Analyzer
smooth muscle antibody
superior mesenteric artery
supplementary motor area

SMA-12

generic term for a battery
of *x* number of blood
chemistry determinations

SMAF

specific macrophage
arming factor

SMAST

Short Michigan Alcoholism
Screening Test

SMBV

suckling mouse brain
vaccine

SMC

selenomethylnorchol-
esterol
single mixing coil

SMO

Senior Medical Officer

SMON

subacute myelo-
opticoneuropathy

SMP

slow-moving protease

SMR

somnolent metabolic rate
standard morbidity ratio
standard mortality ratio
submucous resection

SMRR

submucous resection and
rhinoplasty

SMX

sulfamethoxazole

SN
serum-neutralizing
student nurse
suprasternal notch

S.N.
L. secundum naturam
(according to nature)

S/N
signal-to-noise ratio

Sn
tin (L. stannum)

SNB
scalene node biopsy

SNF
skilled nursing facility

SNHL
sensorineural hearing loss

SNIVT
Society of Non-Invasive
Vascular Technology

SNM
Society of Nuclear
Medicine

SNM-TS
Society of Nuclear
Medicine—Technologists
Section

SNOP
Systematized
Nomenclature of
Pathology

SNR
signal-to-noise ratio

SNS
sympathetic nervous
system

SO
salpingo-oophorectomy
spheno-occipital
synchondrosis

SO *(continued)*
stitches out
superior oblique
sutures out

SOAP
Subjective, Objective,
Assessment, Plan

SOB
shortness of breath

SOBE
short of breath w/exertion

SOC
sequential-type oral
contraceptive

soc
society

SODAS
spheroidal oral drug
absorption system

SOL
space-occupying lesion

Sol.
solution

sol
soluble

solidif
solidifies

soln
solution

solv.
L. solve (dissolve)

soly
solubility

SOM
secretory otitis media
serous otitis media

SOMI
sternal-occipital-
mandibular immobilizer

SOP

standard operating
procedure

S. op. s.

L. si opus sit (if it is
necessary)

S.O.S.

L. si opus sit (if it is
necessary)

SOTT

synthetic medium old
tuberculin trichloroacetic
acid (precipitated)

SP

sacrum to pubis
shunt procedure
sinus pause
skin potential
spine
status post
steady potential
suicide precautions
summating potential
suprapubic
symphysis pubis
systolic pressure

S/P

status post

2-S P

transport medium used for
mycoplasma isolation

sp

species
specific
sperm
spine
spleen

sp.

L. spiritus (spirit)

s/p

status post

SPA

single photon
absorptiometry
suprapubic aspiration

SPAI

steroid protein activity
index

SPBI

serum protein-bound
iodine

SPC

saturated
phosphatidylcholine
concentration

SPCA

serum prothrombin
conversion accelerator
(blood coagulation factor
VII)

sp cd

spinal cord

SPE

serum protein
electrophoresis

SPEC

specimen

spec

specimen
spectroscopy

SPECT

single photon emission
computed tomography

SPF

specific pathogen–free
split products of fibrin
sun protection factor

sp fl

spinal fluid

sp gr

specific gravity

SPH
> secondary pulmonary hemosiderosis

Sph
> sphingosine

sph
> spherical
> spherical lens

SPHE
> Society of Public Health Educators

SPI
> serum precipitable iodine

spir.
> L. spiritus (spirit)

SPL
> sound pressure level
> spontaneous lesion

spm
> a gene that leads to suppression and mutation of mutants that are unstable

spont
> spontaneous

SPP
> suprapubic prostatectomy

spp
> plural of sp (species)
> subspecies

SPRINT
> Special Psychiatric Rapid Intervention Team

SPS
> sodium polyanetholsulfonate
> sulfite polymyxin
> sulfadiazine

SPSS
> Statistical Package for the Social Sciences

Spt.
> L. spiritus (spirit)

SPTA
> spatial peak temporal average

SQ
> subcutaneous

sq
> square

sq. cm.
> square centimeter

sqq
> L. sequentia (and following)

SQUID
> superconducting quantum-interference device

SR
> secretion rate
> sedimentation rate
> sensitization response
> side rails
> sigma reaction
> sinus rhythm
> skin resistance
> stimulation ratio
> superior rectus
> systemic resistance
> system review

Sr
> strontium

sr
> steradian

SRBC
> sheep red blood cells

SRC
> sedimented red cells
> sheep red cells

SRF
> skin reactive factor

SRF *(continued)*
> somatotropin releasing factor
> split renal function
> subretinal fluid

SRF-A
> slow-reacting factor of anaphylaxis

SRFS
> split renal function study

SRH
> somatotropin releasing hormone

SRIF
> somatostatin

SRM
> Standard Reference Materials

SRN
> State Registered Nurse (England and Wales)

sRNA
> soluble ribonucleic acid

SRS
> slow-reacting substance

SRS-A
> slow reacting substance of anaphylaxis

SRT
> sedimentation rate test
> speech reception threshold

SRY
> sex-determining region Y

SS
> saliva sample
> *Salmonella-Shigella*
> saturated solution
> soapsuds
> somatostatin
> statistically significant
> subaortic stenosis
> supersaturated

ss
> single stranded

ss.
> L. semis (one half)

s/s
> signs and symptoms

SSA
> salicylsalicylic acid
> skin-sensitizing antibody
> Social Security Administration
> sulfosalicylic acid test

SSD
> source-skin distance
> sum of square deviations

ssDNA
> single-stranded DNA

SSE
> soapsuds enema

SSEP
> somatosensory evoked potential

SSI
> Social Security Income

SSKI
> saturated solution of potassium iodide

SSM
> superficial spreading melanoma

SSN
> severely subnormal

SSP
> Sanarelli-Shwartzman phenomenon
> subacute sclerosing panencephalitis

SSPE
> subacute sclerosing panencephalitis

ssRNA
single-stranded RNA

SSS
scalded skin syndrome
sick sinus syndrome
specific soluble substance
sterile saline soak

s.s.s.
L. stratum super stratum
(layer upon layer)

SSU
sterile supply unit

SSV
simian sarcoma virus

S.S.V.
L. sub signo veneni (under
a poison label)

S&Sx
signs and symptoms

ST
esotropic
sinus tachycardia
skin test
slight trace
smokeless tobacco
sore throat
stable toxin
standardized test
sternothyroid
stomach
subtalar
subtotal
surface tension
survival time

St
stoke

St.
L. stet (let it stand)

st
straight

STA
serum thrombotic
accelerator

stab
stab cell
stab neutrophil

STA-MCA
superficial temporal artery
to middle cerebral artery

Staph
Staphylococcus

stat.
L. statim (immediately)

STC
soft tissue calcification
subtotal colectomy

STD
sexually transmitted
disease
skin test dose
skin to tumor distance
standard test dose

std
saturated

STEL
short-term exposure limit

stet.
let it stand

STH
somatotropic (growth)
hormone
somatotropin

STI
systolic time intervals

STJ
subtalar joint

STK
streptokinase

STLI
subtotal lymphoid
irradiation

STM
short-term memory

STM *(continued)*
   streptomycin

STP
   standard temperature and
      pressure

STPD
   standard temperature and
      pressure, dry

Strep
   Streptococcus

STS
   sequence-tagged site
   serologic test for syphilis
   Society of Thoracic
      Surgeons
   standard test for syphilis

STSG
   split thickness skin graft

STT
   serial thrombin time

STU
   skin test unit

STVA
   subtotal villose atrophy

STZ
   streptozocin

Stz
   streptozocin

su.
   L. sumat (let him take)

SUA
   serum uric acid
   single umbilical artery

Sub fin. coct.
   L. sub finem coctionis
      (toward the end of
      boiling)

subl
   sublimes

sub q
   subcutaneous

substc
   substance concentration

substfr
   substance fraction

SUD
   sudden unexpected death
   sudden unexplained death

SUDS
   sudden unexplained death
      syndrome

SUID
   sudden unexplained infant
      death

sum.
   L. sumat (let him take)
   L. sumendum (to be taken)

sum. tal.
   L. sumat talem (let him
      take one like this)

SUN
   serum urea nitrogen

SUP
   superior

sup
   superior

supp
   suppository

suppl
   supplement

surg
   surgery
   surgical

SUS
   stained urinary sediment

SUUD
   sudden unexpected,
      unexplained death

SV
    severe
    simian virus
    sinus venosus
    snake venom
    stroke volume
    subclavian vein
    supraventricular
    supravital

S.V.
    L. spiritus vini (alcoholic
      spirit)

SV40
    simian virus 40

Sv
    sievert

SVA
    supraventricular activity

SVAS
    supravalvular aortic
      stenosis

SVB
    supraventricular beats

SVC
    slow vital capacity
    superior vena cava

SVCG
    spatial vectorcardiogram

SVD
    spontaneous vaginal
      delivery
    spontaneous vertex
      delivery

SVG
    saphenous vein graft

SVI
    syncytiovascular
      membrane

SVR
    L. spiritus vini rectificatus
      (rectified alcoholic spirit)

SVR *(continued)*
    systemic vascular
      resistance

SVS
    Society for Vascular
      Surgery

SVT
    L. spiritus vini tenuis
      (proof spirit)
    supraventricular
      tachycardia

SW
    spiral wound
    stab wound
    stroke work

SWD
    short wave diathermy

SWI
    stroke work index

SWOG
    Southwest Oncology Group

SWS
    slow wave sleep

Sx
    signs
    symptoms

sym
    symptoms

sym
    symmetrical

sympt
    symptoms

Synf
    synovial fluid

Syn Fl
    synovial fluid

Syr.
    L. syrupus (syrup)

SZ
    streptozocin

SZ *(continued)*
    streptozotocin
    schizophrenic
    seizure

Sz
    schizophrenic
    seizure

T

intraocular tension
temperature
tera-
terminal (congenital
  absence of limb)
tesla
testis
thoracic vertebra (T1–T12)
thorax
threonine
thymidine
thymine
tight
time
tissue
tocopherol
torque
tritium

2,4,5-T

2,4,5-trichlorophenoxy
  acetic acid

T$^+$

increased intraocular
  tension

T$^-$

decreased intraocular
  tension

T1

longitudinal relaxation
  time

T2

transverse relaxation time

T

Taenia
transmittance
Treponema
Trichophyton
Trypanosoma

T$_1$

tricuspid valve closure

T$_{1/2}$, t$_{1/2}$

half-life
half-time

T$_3$

triiodothyronine

T$_4$

thyroxine

T$_m$

melting temperature
tubular maximum

T$_{max}$

time of maximum
  concentration

T$_{mg}$

maximal tubular
  reabsorption of glucose

T°

temperature

T

testes both down

t

telephoned
temporal
tertiary
test of significance
translocation

t

temperature
time

t$_{1/2}$

half-life
half-time

t$_m$

temperature midpoint
  (Celsius)

τ

mean life
torque

TA
  alkaline tuberculin
  axillary temperature
  therapeutic abortion
  titratable acid
  toxin-antitoxin
  tube agglutination

T&A
  tonsillectomy and
    adenoidectomy

Ta
  tantalum
  tarsus
  tarsal amputation

TAA
  tumor-associated antigen

TAANA
  American Association of
    Nurse Attorneys

TAB vaccine
  typhoid-paratyphoid A and
    B vaccine

tabs
  tablets

TAC
  total abdominal colectomy
  tetracaine, epinephrine,
    and cocaine

TAD
  6-thioguanine, cytarabine,
    and daunorubicin
  thoracic asphyxiant
    dystrophy
  transient acantholytic
    dermatosis

TADAC
  therapeutic abortion,
    dilation, aspiration, and
    curettage

TAF
  albumose-free tuberculin
  toxoid-antitoxin floccules
  trypsin-aldehyde-fuchsin

TAF (continued)
  tumor angiogenic factor

TAH
  total abdominal
    hysterectomy

TAL
  tendo Achillis lengthening
  thymic alymphoplasia

Tal.
  L. talis (such a one)

TAM
  tamoxifen
  toxoid-antitoxin mixture

TAME
  toluene-sulfo-trypsin
    arginine methyl ester

TAO
  thromboangiitis obliterans
  triacetyloleandomycin

TAPVD
  total anomalous
    pulmonary venous
    drainage

TAR
  thrombocytopenia–absent
    radius (syndrome)

TARA
  tumor-associated rejection
    antigen

TAT
  tetanus antitoxin
  thematic apperception test
  thromboplastin activation
    test
  total antitryptic activity
  toxin-antitoxin
  turn-around time
  tyrosine aminotransferase

TATA
  transanal abdominal
    transanal
    proctosigmoidectomy and
    coloanal anastomosis

TB
  terminal bronchiole
  toluidine blue
  total base
  total body
  tracheobronchitis
  tubercle bacillus
  tuberculin
  tuberculosis

Tb
  terbium
  tubercle bacillus

t.b.
  tubercle bacillus

TBA
  tertiary butylacetate
  testosterone-binding
    affinity
  thiobarbituric acid

tbc
  tuberculosis

TBD
  total body density

TBE
  tuberculin bacillin
    emulsion

TBF
  total body fat

TBG
  thyroxine-binding globulin

TBGP
  total blood granulocyte
    pool

TBH
  total body hematocrit

TBI
  thyroxine-binding index
  total body involved
  total body irradiation

TBII
  TSH-binding inhibitory
    immunoglobulin

T bili
  total bilirubin

TBK
  total body potassium

TBLC
  term birth, living child

TBM
  tuberculous meningitis
  tubular basement
    membrane

TBN
  bacillus emulsions

TBP
  thyroxine-binding protein

TBPA
  thyroxine-binding
    prealbumin

TB-Rd
  tuberculosis–respiratory
    disease

TBS
  total body solute
  tribromosalicylanilide
  triethanolamine-buffered
    saline

tbs
  tablespoon

TBSA
  total body surface area

tbsp
  tablespoon

TBT
  tolbutamide test
  tracheobronchial toilet

TBV
  total blood volume

TBW
  total body water
  total body weight

TBX
   whole body irradiation

TC
   taurocholate
   temperature compensation
   tetracycline
   thermal conductivity
   throat culture
   tissue culture
   to contain
   total cholesterol
   transcobalamin
   tuberculin, contagious
   tubocurarine

Tc
   technetium

T&C
   turn and cough
   type and crossmatch

TCA
   tricarboxylic acid
   trichloroacetate
   trichloracetic acid
   tricyclic antidepressant

TCAP
   trimethylcetylammonium
      pentachlorophenate

TCB
   β strep throat culture

TCBS
   thiosulfate citrate bile salts
      sucrose

TCC
   transitional cell carcinoma
   trichlorocarbanilide

TCD
   tissue culture dose
   transcranial Doppler

TCD$_{50}$
   median tissue culture dose

TCDB
   turn, cough, and deep
      breath

TCDD
   2,3,7,8-tetrachlorodibenzo-
      para-dioxin

TCE
   trichloroethylene

T cell
   thymus-derived cell

TCF
   total coronary flow

TCG
   time compensation gain

TCH
   total circulating
      hemoglobin
   turn, cough, and
      hyperventilate

TCI
   to come in
   transient cerebral ischemia

TCi
   tetracurie

TCID
   tissue culture infective
      dose

TCID$_{50}$
   median tissue culture
      infective dose

TCIE
   transient cerebral ischemic
      episode

TCM
   tissue culture media

TCMA
   transcortical motor
      aphasia

TCMI
   T cell–mediated immunity

TCNS
   transcutaneous nerve
      stimulator

TCO
> total contact orthosis

TCOM
> transcutaneous oximetry

TCP
> tricalcium phosphate
> tricresyl phosphate

TcPO$_2$
> transcutaneous oxygen
> pressure

TCR
> T cell antigen receptor

tcRNA
> translation control RNA

TCSA
> tetrachlorosalicylanilide

TCT
> thrombin clotting time
> thyrocalcitonin

TD
> tetanus-diphtheria toxoid
> (pediatric use)
> thoracic duct
> threshold of discomfort
> thymus-dependent
> to deliver
> torsion dystonia
> transverse diameter
> treatment discontinued

Td
> tetanus and diphtheria
> toxoids adult type

TD$_{50}$
> median toxic dose

TDA
> TSH-displacing antibody

TDE
> tetrachlorodiphenylethane

TDF
> thoracic duct fistula
> thoracic duct flow

TDI
> toluene diisocyanate
> total-dose infusion

TDL
> thoracic duct lymph

TDM
> therapeutic drug
> monitoring

tDNA
> transfer-DNA

TDP
> thoracic duct pressure
> ribothymidine
> 5′-diphosphate

TDS
> total dissolved solids

t.d.s.
> L. ter die sumendum (to be
> taken three times a day)

TDT
> tumor doubling time

TdT
> terminal deoxynucleotidyl
> transferase

TE
> threshold energy
> tissue-equivalent
> total estrogen (excretion)
> tracheoesophageal

TE$_A$
> total error goal

Te
> tetanic contraction
> tellurium
> tetanus

TEA
> tetraethylammonium

TEAC
> tetraethylammonium
> chloride

TEAE cellulose
  triethylaminoethyl
    cellulose

TeBG
  testosterone-estradiol–
    binding globulin

T&EC
  trauma and emergency
    center

tech
  technical

TED
  threshold erythema dose
  thromboembolic disease

TEDD
  total end-diastolic
    diameter

TEE
  transesophageal
    echocardiography
  tyrosine ethyl ester

TEF
  tracheoesophageal fistula

TEG
  thromboelastogram

TEIB
  triethyleneiminobenzo
    quinone

TEL
  tetraethyl acid

TEM
  transmission electron
    microscope
  triethylenemelamine

TEMP
  temperature

temp. dext.
  L. tempori dextro (to the
    right temple)

temp. sinist.
  L. tempori sinistro (to the
    left temple)

TEN
  toxic epidermal necrolysis

TENS
  transcutaneous electrical
    nerve stimulation

TEP
  thromboendophlebectomy

TEPA
  triethylenephosphoramide

TEPP
  tetraethyl pyrophosphate

tert
  tertiary

TES
  trimethylaminoethane-
    sulfonic acid

TESD
  total end-systolic diameter

TET
  treadmill exercise test

Tet
  tetanus
  tetralogy of Fallot

TETD
  tetraethylthiuram disulfide

TEV
  talipes equinovarus

TF
  tactile fremitus
  tetralogy of Fallot
  thymol flocculation
  tissue-damaging factor
  to follow
  transfer factor
  tuberculin filtrate
  tubular fluid

TFA
    total fatty acids

TFE
    polytetrafluoroethylene
    tetrafluoroethylene

TFL
    tensor fasciae latae

Tfm
    testicular feminization
    syndrome

TFS
    testicular feminization
    syndrome

TG
    tendon graft
    thioguanine
    thyroglobulin
    toxic goiter
    triglyceride

Tg
    thioguanine

t$\dot{\gamma}$
    shear rate

TGA
    thyroglobulin antibodies
    transposition of the great
    arteries

TGAR
    total graft area rejected

TGC
    time gain compensation
    time-varied gain control

TGE
    transmissible
    gastroenteritis of swine

TGF
    transforming growth factor

TGFA
    triglyceride fatty acid

TGL
    triglyceride

TGL *(continued)*
    triglyceride lipase

TGT
    thromboplastin generation
    test
    thromboplastin generation
    time

TGV
    thoracic gas volume
    transposition of the great
    vessels

TH
    thoracic
    thyrohyoid
    thyroid hormone

Th
    thigh
    thigh amputation
    thorium

th
    thoracic

THA
    total hip arthroplasty
    total hydroxyapatite

THAM
    tris(hydroxymethyl)amino-
    methane

THC
    tetrahydrocannabinol

Δ9 THC
    delta-9-tetrahydrocannabin-
    ol

Thd
    ribothymidine

THDOC
    tetrahydrodeoxycortico-
    sterone

THE
    tetrahydrocortisone

TITh
    3,5,3′-triiodothyronine

THF
    humoral thymic factor
    tetrahydrofolate
    tetrahydrofolic acid
    tetrahydrofuran

THFA
    tetrahydrofolic acid

THO
    Thogoto orthomyxovirus
    titrated water

THP
    total hydroxyproline

THR
    total hip replacement

Thr
    threonine

THS
    tetrahydro-compound S

Thy
    thymine

THz
    tetrahertz

TI
    thoracic index
    tibia, complete (congenital
      absence of limb)
    time interval
    total ion
    transverse inlet
    tricuspid incompetence
    tricuspid insufficiency

Ti
    titanium

TIA
    transient ischemic attack

ti
    tibia, incomplete
      (congenital absence of
      limb)

TIBC
    total iron-binding capacity

TIBO
    tetrahydroimidazobenzo-
      diazepinone

TIC
    trypsin-inhibitory capacity

TID
    titrated initial dose

t.i.d.
    L. ter in die (three times a
      day)

TIE
    transient ischemic episode

TIG
    tetanus immune globulin

TIMI
    Thrombolysis in
      Myocardial Infarction
      Study Group

TIN
    tubulointerstitial
      nephropathy

t.i.n.
    L. ter in nocte (three times
      a night)

tinct.
    tinctura
    tincture

TIS
    tumor in situ

TISS
    Therapeutic Intervention
      Scoring System

TIT
    Treponema immobilization
      test
    triiodothyronine

TIV
    trivalent inactivated
      influenza vaccine

TIVC
thoracic inferior vena cava

TJ
tendon jerk
triceps jerk

TJR
total joint replacement

TK
thymidine kinase

TKA
transketolase activity

TKD
tokodynamometer

TKG
tokodynagraph

TKO
to keep open

TKR
total knee replacement

TL
temporal lobe
total lipids
tubal ligation

Tl
thallium

TLA
translumbar aortogram

TLC
tender loving care
thin-layer chromatography
total L-chain concentration
total lung capacity
total lung compliance

TLD
thermoluminescent
dosimeter
tumor lethal dose

T/LD$_{100}$
minimum dose causing
death or malformation of
100 per cent of fetuses

TLE
thin-layer electrophoresis

TLI
total lymphoid irradiation

TLiSA1
T lineage-specific
activation antigen 1

TLSO
thoracolumbosacral
orthosis

TLV
threshold limit value
total lung volume

TM
temporomandibular
trademark
transmetatarsal
tympanic membrane

Tm
thulium
transport maximum

TMA
trimethoxyamphetamine

TmG
maximal tubular
reabsorption of glucose

TMI
transmandibular implant

TMIF
tumor cell migration
inhibition factor

TMJ
temporomandibular joint
temporomandibular joint
dysfunction

TMJS
temporomandibular joint
syndrome

TML
tetramethyl lead

TMN
> tumor-node-metastasis

TMP
> ribothymidylic acid
> thymidine
> 5′-monophosphate
> thymine ribonucleoside
> phosphate
> thymolphthalein
> monophosphate
> trimethoprim

TMP/SMX
> trimethoprim-sulfamethoxa-
> zole

TMST
> treadmill stress test

TMT
> tarsometatarsal

TMTD
> tetramethylthiuram
> disulfide

TMV
> tobacco mosaic virus

Tn
> normal intraocular tension
> thoron

TNCC
> trauma nursing core
> course

TNF
> tumor necrosis factor

TNI
> total nodal irradiation

TNM
> tumor-node-metastasis

TNP
> trinitrophenyl

TNS
> transcutaneous nerve
> stimulation

TNT
> trinitrotoluene

TNTC
> too numerous to count
> (cells in urinalysis)

TO
> original tuberculin
> telephone order
> tincture of opium
> tubo-ovarian

TOA
> tubo-ovarian abscess

TOCP
> triorthocresyl phosphate

tomo
> tomogram

TOP
> termination of pregnancy

TOPV
> poliovirus vaccine live oral
> trivalent

TORCH
> toxoplasmosis, other
> infections, rubella,
> cytomegalovirus
> infection, and herpes
> simplex

TORP
> total ossicular replacement
> prosthesis

TOS
> thoracic outlet syndrome

tox
> toxicity
> toxicology

TP
> posterior tibial
> temperature and pressure
> threshold potential
> thrombocytopenic purpura
> total protein

TP *(continued)*
    tryptophan
    tube precipitin
    tuberculin precipitation

TPA
    Treponema pallidum
      agglutination
    tissue plasminogen
      activator

t-PA
    tissue plasminogen
      activator

TPAG
    total protein and
      albumin/globulin

TPBF
    total pulmonary blood flow

TPC
    thromboplastic plasma
      component
    total proctocolectomy

TPCF
    Treponema pallidum
      complement fixation

TPG
    transplacental gradient

TPH
    transplacental hemorrhage

TPHA
    Treponema pallidum
      hemagglutination assay

TPI
    Treponema pallidum
      immobilization
    treponemal immobilization
      test (cardiolipin)
    triose phosphate isomerase

TPIA
    Treponema pallidum
      immobilization adherence

TPM
    temporary pacemaker

TPM *(continued)*
    triphenylmethane

TPN
    total parenteral nutrition
    triphosphopyridine
      nucleotide

TPNH
    reduced
      triphosphopyridine
      nucleotide

TPP
    thiamine pyrophosphate

TPPN
    total peripheral parenteral
      nutrition

TPR
    temperature, pulse, and
      respiration
    testosterone production
      rate
    total peripheral resistance
    total pulmonary resistance

TPS
    tumor polysaccharide
      substance

TPT
    typhoid-paratyphoid
      (vaccine)

TPTZ
    tripyridyltriazine

TPVR
    total pulmonary vascular
      resistance

TQ
    Fagerstrom Tolerance
      Scale
    tocopherolquinone

TR
    (certificate in) therapeutic
      radiology
    tetrazolium reduction
    total resistance
    total response

TR *(continued)*
    tricuspid regurgitation
    tuberculin residue

Tr
    trace

tr
    L. tinctura
    tincture

TRA
    transaldolase

trach
    tracheostomy

TRBF
    total renal blood flow

TRC
    tanned red cells
    total ridge count

TRF
    thyrotropin releasing
        factor
    T-cell replacing factor

TRH
    thyrotropin releasing
        hormone

TRI
    tetrazolium reduction
        inhibition

TRIC
    trachoma inclusion
        conjunctivitis (group of
        organisms)

Trid.
    L. triduum (three days)

Trig
    triglycerides

TRIS
    tris(hydroxymethyl)amino-
        methane

Tris
    tris(hydroxymethyl)amino-
        methane

Trit.
    L. tritura (triturate)

TRK
    transketolase

TRMC
    tetramethylrhodamino-
        isothiocyanate

tRNA
    transfer RNA

TRNG
    tetracycline-resistant
        Neisseria gonorrhoeae

troch.
    trochiscus

TRP
    tubular reabsorption of
        phosphorus (phosphate)

Trp
    tryptophan

TRPT
    theoretical renal
        phosphorus threshold

TRU
    turbidity reducing unit

T$_3$RU
    triiodothyronine resin
        uptake

Try
    former abbreviation for
        tryptophan

TS
    test solution
    transsexual
    tricuspid stenosis
    temperature sensitive
    tropical sprue

T&S
    type and screen

ts
    temperature sensitive

TSA
        total shoulder arthroplasty
        trypticase soy agar
        tumor-specific antigen

T₄SA
        thyroxine-specific activity

TSB
        trypticase soy broth

TSC
        technetium sulfur colloid
        thiosemicarbizide

TSD
        target skin distance
        Tay-Sachs disease

TSE
        testicular self-examination
        trisodium edetate

TSF
        tissue-coding factor
        triceps skinfold

TSH
        thyroid-stimulating
            hormone

TSH-RF
        thyroid-stimulating
            hormone–releasing factor

TSI
        thyroid-stimulating
            immunoglobulins
        triple sugar iron (agar)

TSP
        total serum protein
        trisodium phosphate
        tropical spastic paraparesis

tsp
        teaspoon

TSPAP
        total serum prostatic acid
            phosphatase

T-spine
        thoracic spine

TSR
        thyroid-to-serum ratio

TSS
        toxic shock syndrome
        tropical splenomegaly
            syndrome

TST
        tumor skin test

TSTA
        tumor-specific
            transplantation antigen

TSY
        trypticase soy yeast

TT
        tetanus toxoid
        tetrazol
        thrombin time
        thymol turbidity
        tilt table
        toilet tissue
        total thyroxine
        transthoracic

TTA
        tetracyclic antidepressants

TTAP
        threaded titanium
            acetabular prosthesis

TTC
        triphenyltetrazolium
            chloride

TTD
        tissue tolerance dose

TTH
        thyrotropic hormone
        tritiated thymidine

TTI
        tension-time index

TTP
        ribothymidine
            5′-triphosphate

TTP *(continued)*
   thrombotic
      thrombocytopenic
      purpura

TTS
   temporary threshold shift

TTT
   tolbutamide tolerance test

TU
   thiouracil
   Todd units
   toxic unit
   tuberculin unit

tuberc
   tuberculosis
   tuberculous

TUR
   transurethral resection

TURBT
   transurethral resection of
      bladder tumor

TURP
   transurethral prostatic
      resection

tus.
   L. tussis (a cough)

TV
   tidal volume
   trial visit
   Trichomonas vaginitis
   tuberculin volutin

TVC
   timed vital capacity
   total volume capacity
   transvaginal cone
   triple voiding cystogram

TVF
   tactile vocal fremitus

TVG
   time-varied gain

TVH
   total vaginal hysterectomy

TVU
   total volume urine

TW
   tap water

TWA
   time-weighted average

TWE
   tap water enema

TWiST
   time without symptoms of
      toxicity

TWL
   transepidermal water loss

TWZ
   triangular working zone

TX
   individual thromboxanes,
      designated by capital
      letters with subscripts
      indicating structural
      features
   traction
   transplant
   treatment

T&X
   type and crossmatch

TXA$_2$
   thromboxane A$_2$

TXB$_2$
   thromboxane B$_2$

TXN
   traction

Ty
   typhoid

Tyr
   tyrosine

TZ
   tuberculin zymoplastiche

U
   international unit (of
      enzyme activity)
   ulna, complete (congenital
      absence of limb)
   unit
   uracil
   uranium
   uridine
   urine

U
   unknown

u
   atomic mass unit
   ulna, incomplete
      (congenital absence of
      limb)

UA
   umbilical artery
   unaggregated
   uric acid
   urinalysis
   urinanalysis
   uterine aspiration

UB
   ultimobranchial body

UBBC
   unsaturated vitamin
      B_{12} –binding capacity

UBF
   uterine blood flow

UBG
   urobilinogen

UBI
   ultraviolet blood
      irradiation

UC
   ulcerative colitis
   ultracentrifugal
   urea clearance
   urethral catheterization

UC *(continued)*
   uterine contractions

U&C
   usual and customary

UCD
   usual childhood diseases

UCG
   urinary chorionic
      gonadotropin

UCHD
   usual childhood diseases

UCI
   urinary (urethral) catheter
      in

UCO
   urinary (urethral) catheter
      out

UCP
   urinary coproporphyrin

UCR
   unconditioned response
   usual, customary, and
      reasonable

UCS
   unconscious

ucs
   unconscious

UD
   urethral discharge
   uroporphyrinogen
      decarboxylase

UDC
   usual diseases of childhood

UDP
   uridine diphosphate

UDPG
   uridine diphosphate
      glucose

UDPGA
    uridine diphosphoglucuronic acid

UDPGal
    uridine diphosphogalactose

UDPGlc
    uridine diphosphoglucose

UDPGT
    uridine diphosphoglycyronyl transferase

UE
    upper extremity

UES
    upper esophageal sphincter

UFA
    unesterified fatty acids

UG
    urogenital

UGDP
    University Group Diabetes Program

UGI
    upper gastrointestinal

UI
    uroporphyrin isomerase

UIBC
    unsaturated iron-binding capacity

UICC
    Union Internationale Contre Cancer
    International Union Against Cancer

UIF
    undegraded insulin factor

UIP
    usual interstitial pneumonitis

UIQ
    upper inner quadrant

UK
    United Kingdom
    unknown
    urokinase

UL
    undifferentiated lymphoma
    upper lobe

U&L
    upper and lower

ULN
    upper limits of normal

ULQ
    upper left quadrant

ult. praes.
    L. ultimum praescriptus (last prescribed)

UM
    unmarried
    uracil mustard

Umb
    umbelliferyl

UMLS
    Unified Medical Language System

UMP
    uridine monophosphate

UN
    ulnar nerve
    urea nitrogen

U:N
    upper limits of normal

uncor
    uncorrected

UNESCO
United Nations
Educational, Scientific,
and Cultural
Organization

ung.
L. unguentum (ointment)

UNICEF
United Nations
International Children's
Emergency Fund

univ
university

UNK
unknown

unk
unknown

UNRRA
United Nations Relief and
Rehabilitation
Organization

uns-
asymmetrical

unsym-
asymmetrical

UO
ureteral orifice
urinary output

UOQ
upper outer quadrant

UOS
units of service

Uosm
urinary osmolality

UP
ureteropelvic
uroporphyrin

U/P
urine-plasma ratio

UPG
uroporphyrinogen

UPI
uteroplacental
insufficiency

UPJ
ureteropelvic junction

UPOR
usual place of residence

UPP
urethral pressure profile

UQ
upper quadrant

UR
unconditioned response
upper respiratory
urine
utilization review

Ura
uracil

URD
upper respiratory disease

Urd
uridine

URF
unidentified reading frame

URI
upper respiratory infection

URIS
upper respiratory
infections

urol
urology

URQ
upper right quadrant

URT
upper respiratory tract

URTI
   upper respiratory tract
   infection

US
   ultrasonic
   ultrasound

U/S
   ultrasound

USAEC
   United States Atomic
   Energy Commission

USAN
   United States Adopted
   Names

USD
   United States Dispensary

USDA
   United States Department
   of Agriculture

USN
   ultrasonic nebulizer

USNRP
   United States National
   Reference Preparation

USO
   unilateral
   salpingo-oophorectomy

USP
   United States
   Pharmacopeia

USPC
   United States
   Pharmacopeial
   Convention

USPHS
   United States Public
   Health Service

USR
   unheated serum reagin
   (test)

Ut
   uterus

UTBG
   unbound thyroxine-binding
   globulin

UTD
   up-to-date

Ut dict.
   L. ut dictum (as directed)

Utend.
   L. utendus (to be used)

UTI
   urinary tract infection

UTP
   uridine triphosphate

UU
   urine urobilinogen

UUN
   urine urea nitrogen

UV
   ultraviolet
   umbilical vein
   urinary volume

UVA
   long-wave ultraviolet
   radiation
   ultraviolet A

UVB
   ultraviolet B

UVC
   ultraviolet C

UVEB
   unifocal ventricular ectopic
   beat

UVJ
   ureterovesical junction

UVL
   ultraviolet light

UVR
   ultraviolet radiation

V

    valine
    vanadium
    vein
    velocity
    ventilation
    volt
    voltage
    volume
    vomiting

V

    Vibrio
    vision
    visual acuity
    voltage
    volume

V_A

    alveolar ventilation

V_{CO}

    carbon monoxide
    (endogenous production)

V_D

    volume dead air space

V_d

    apparent volume of
    distribution (V area)

V_E

    minute volume (expired)

$\dot{V}_E$

    minute ventilation

V_{max}

    maximum velocity of an
    enzyme-catalyzed
    reaction

V_T

    tidal volume

$\dot{V}$

    gas flow, frequently with
    subscripts indicating

$\dot{V}$ *(continued)*

    location and chemical
    species
    ventilation, frequently
    with subscript

v

    venous
    volt

v.

    L. vena (vein)

υ

    velocity
    voltage

$\bar{v}$

    as a subscript, refers to
    mixed venous

VA

    vacuum aspiration
    ventricular arrest
    ventriculoatrial
    vertebral artery
    Veterans Administration
    visual acuity
    visual discriminatory
    acuity
    volt-ampere

V-A

    ventriculoatrial

Va

    alveolar ventilation

VAB-6

    vinblastine, dactinomycin,
    bleomycin, cisplatin,
    cyclophosphamide

VABCD

    vinblastine, doxorubicin,
    dacarbazine, lomustine,
    and bleomycin sulfate

VAC
> vincristine, dactinomycin, and cyclophosphamide

VACTERL
> vertebral, anal, cardiac, tracheal, esophageal, renal, and limb

VAD
> venous access device
> ventricular assist device
> vincristine, doxorubicin, and dexamethasone

vag.
> vagina

Val
> valine

VALE
> visual acuity, left eye

VALG
> Veterans Administration Lung Cancer Study Group

VAMP
> vincristine, prednisone, methotrexate

$\dot{V}a/Q$
> ventilation/perfusion ratio

VAR
> variant

var.
> variant
> variety

VARE
> visual acuity, right eye

VASAG
> Veterans Administration Surgical Adjuvant Cancer Chemotherapy Study Group

VASC
> vascular

VASC *(continued)*
> Verbal Auditory Screen for Children
> Visual-Auditory Screen Test for Children

vasc
> vascular

VAT
> Veterinary Aptitude/Admission Test
> atrial synchronous ventricular (pacemaker code)

VATER
> vertebral defects, anal atresia, tracheo-esophageal fistula with esophageal atresia, and radial and renal anomalies

VB
> vinblastine
> ventricular bradycardia

VBAP
> vincristine, carmustine, doxorubicin, and prednisone

VBL
> vinblastine

Vbl
> vinblastine

VBM
> vinblastine, bleomycin sulfate, and methotrexate

VBP
> vinblastine, bleomycin, and cisplatin

VBS
> veronal-buffered saline

VBS:FBS
> veronal-buffered saline:fetal bovine serum

VC
pulmonary capillary blood
volume
vena cava
ventilatory capacity
vincristine
vital capacity
vocal cords

VCA
viral capsid antigen

VCE
vagina ectocervix and
endocervix (smear)

VCG
vectorcardiogram

VCR
vincristine sulfate

Vcr
vincristine

VCT
venous clotting time

VCU
voiding cystourethogram

VCUG
voiding cystourethrogram
vapor density

VD
venereal disease

Vd
volume dead air space
volume of distribution

VDA
visual discriminatory
acuity

VDBR
volume of distribution of
bilirubin

VDD
atrial synchronous
ventricular inhibited

VDDR
vitamin D–dependent
rickets

VDEL
Venereal Disease
Experimental Laboratory

VDG
venereal
disease—gonorrhea

vdg
voiding

VDH
valvular disease of the
heart
vascular disease of the
heart

VDL
visual detection level

VDM
vasodepressor material

VDP
vincristine, daunorubicin,
and prednisone

VDRL
Venereal Disease Research
Laboratories

VDRR
vitamin D–resistant rickets

VDS
venereal disease—syphilis

VE
vaginal examination
ventricular ectopic(s)
visual efficiency
volumic ejection

V&E
Vinethene and ether

VEA
ventricular ectopic activity

VEB
    ventricular ectopic beats

VEE
    Venezuelan equine
        encephalomyelitis

VEE virus
    Venezuelan equine
        encephalomyelitis virus

VEM
    vasoexcitor material

VENT
    ventral
    ventricular

vent
    ventral
    ventricular

VEP
    visual evoked potential

VER
    visual evoked response

VES
    bladder
    vesicular

Vesic.
    vesicatorium (a blister)
    L. vesicula (a blister)

VESV
    vesicular exanthema of
        swine virus

VET
    veteran

Vet
    veteran

VF
    ventricular fibrillation
    ventricular fluid
    visual field
    vocal fremitus

vf
    field of vision
    visual field

Vfib
    ventricular fibrillation

VFL
    ventricular flutter

VFP
    ventricular fluid pressure

VG
    ventricular gallop

VGH
    very good health

VH
    vaginal hysterectomy
    venous hematocrit
    viral hepatitis

VHD
    valvular heart disease
    viral hematodepressive
        disease

VHDL
    very high density
        lipoprotein

VHSV
    viral hemorrhagic
        septicemia

VI
    valgus index
    volume index

VIA
    virus-inactivating agent

vib
    vibration

VIG
    vaccinia immune globulin

VIN
    L. vinum (wine)

VIP
>vasoactive intestinal
>polypeptide
>very important patient
>voluntary interruption of
>pregnancy

VIS
>vaginal irrigation smear

VISI
>volar-flexed intercalated
>segment instability

vit
>vitamin
>vital capacity

vit. ov. sol.
>L. vitello ovi solutus
>(dissolved in yolk of egg)

viz.
>L. videlicet (namely)

VLA
>very late antigen

VLBW
>very low birth weight

VLCD
>very low calorie diet

VLDL
>very low density
>lipoprotein

V lead
>voltage lead

VLSI
>very large scale integration

VM
>ventricular muscle
>viomycin
>voltmeter

VMA
>vanillylmandelic acid

VMC
>void metal composite

VMCP
>vincristine, melphalan,
>cyclophosphamide, and
>prednisone

VMD
>L. Veterinariae Medicinae
>Doctor (Doctor of
>Veterinary Medicine)

VMF
>etoposide, methotrexate,
>fluorouracil

VMH
>ventromedial
>hypothalamic

V-MI
>Volpe-Manhold Index

VMR
>vasomotor rhinitis

VN
>virus-neutralizing
>visiting nurse

VNA
>Visiting Nurse Association

VNR
>vitronectin receptor (VNR)

VO
>verbal order

VO$_2$
>oxygen consumption

VOD
>venous occlusive disease

V.O.D.
>L. visio oculus dextra
>(vision, right eye)

vol
>volume
>voluntary

volfr
>volume fraction

VOM
volt-ohm-milliammeter

VOO
ventricular asynchronous (pacemaker code)

V.O.S.
L. visio oculus sinister (vision, left eye)

v. o. s.
L. vitello ovi solutus (dissolved in yolk)

V.O.U.
L. visio oculus uterque (vision, each eye)

VP
variegate porphyria
vasopressin
venipuncture
venous pressure
ventricular pause
vindesine, cisplatin
Voges-Proskauer (reaction)

VP-16
etoposide

Vp-16
etoposide

V&P
vagotomy and pyloroplasty

VPB
ventricular premature beat

VPC
vapor-phase chromatography
ventricular premature contraction
ventricular premature complex
volume of packed cells
volume per cent

VPD
ventricular premature depolarization

VPF
vascular permeability factor

VPL
ventroposterolateral

VPRC
volume of packed red cells

VPS
Volume Performance Standards

VP test
Voges-Proskauer test

VQ
ventilation-perfusion

VQE
Visa Qualifying Exam

VQ scan
ventilation quantitation imaging technique

VR
valve replacement
vascular resistance
venous return
ventilation ratio
vocal resonance
vocational rehabilitation

VRBC
red blood cell volume

V region
variable region

VRI
viral respiratory infection

VS
venisection
ventricular septum
vital signs
volumetric solution

vs
versus

v.s.
    vibration seconds

VSD
    ventricular septal defect

VSG
    variable surface
        glycoprotein

VSL
    very serious list

VSOK
    vital signs normal

VSS
    vital signs stable

VSV
    vesicular stomatitis virus

VSW
    ventricular stroke work

VT
    tidal volume
    vacuum tuberculin
    ventricular tachycardia

V&T
    volume and tension

VTach
    ventricular tachycardia

VTE
    venous thromboembolism

VU
    volume unit

VUR
    vesico-ureteric reflux

VV
    varicose veins
    viper venom

VV *(continued)*
    vulva and vagina

V&V
    vulva and vagina

$V_D V_T$
    physiologic dead space in
        percent of tidal volume

vv.
    L. venae (veins)

v/v
    volume (of solute) per
        volume (of solvent)

VVI
    ventricular demand
        inhibited (pacemaker
        code)

V/VI
    grade 5 on a 6-grade basis

VVs
    varicose veins

VVT
    ventricular demand
        triggered (pacemaker
        code)

VW
    vessel wall

vWf
    von Willebrand's factor

VZ
    varicella-zoster

VZIG
    varicella-zoster immune
        globulin

VZV
    varicella zoster virus

W

W
- tungsten
- watch the finding
- water
- week
- wehnelt (unit of roentgen ray penetrating ability)
- weight
- well closed
- white
- widowed
- wife
- with

W
- work

W+
- weakly positive

w
- week
- weight
- white
- widow
- widowed
- widower
- wife
- with

WA
- when awake

WAIS
- Wechsler Adult Intelligence Scale

WAP
- wandering atrial pacemaker

WAR
- whole abdominal radiotherapy

WASP
- World Association of Societies of Pathology

WB
- weight bearing
- whole blood
- whole body
- Willowbrook (virus)

Wb
- weber

WBAT
- weight bearing as tolerated

WBC
- white blood cell
- white blood (cell) count

wbc
- white blood cell

WBC/hpf
- white blood cells per high power field

WBF
- whole blood folate

WBGT
- wet bulb globe temperature

WBH
- whole blood hematocrit

WBR
- whole body radiation

WBS
- whole body scan

WC
- water closet
- wheelchair
- white cell
- white cell casts
- whooping cough

WC'
- whole complement

wc
- wheelchair

w/c
  wheelchair

WCC
  white cell count

WCSG
  Western Cancer Study
    Group

WD
  wallerian degeneration
  well developed
  well differentiated
  wet dressing

W4D
  Worth four-dot (test)

WDHA
  watery diarrhea with
    hypokalemic alkalosis

WDLL
  well-differentiated
    lymphocytic lymphoma

WDS
  wavelength-dispersive
    x-ray spectrometry

WDWN
  well developed, well
    nourished

WE
  western encephalitis
  western encephalomyelitis

WEE
  western equine
    encephalitis
  western equine
    encephalomyelitis

WEE virus
  western equine
    encephalomyelitis virus

WEST
  work evaluation systems
    technology

WF
  Weil-Felix (reaction)
  white female

WFE
  Williams flexion exercises

WFR
  Weil-Felix reaction

WGA
  wheat germ agglutinin

WHA
  World Health Assembly

WHO
  World Health Organization
  WHO histologic
    classification of ovarian
    tumors

WHR
  ratio of waist to hip
    circumference

WHVP
  wedged hepatic venous
    pressure

WIA
  wounded in action

WID
  widow
  widower

wid
  widow
  widower

WISC
  Wechsler Intelligence
    Scale Children

WK
  Wernicke-Korsakoff
    (syndrome)

wk
  weak
  week
  work

WL
waiting list

wl
wavelength

WLT
waterload test

WM
white male

WMA
wall motion abnormality
World Medical Association

WMR
work metabolic rate

Wms flex ex
Williams flexion exercises

WMX
whirlpool, massage, and
exercise

WN
well nourished

WNL
within normal limits

WO
written order

W/O
water in oil
without

w/o
without

WP
weakly positive
whirlpool

WPB
whirlpool bath

WPW
Wolff-Parkinson-White
(syndrome)

WR
Wasserman reaction
weakly reactive
wrist

Wr^a
Wright antigen

wr
wrist

WRAT
Wide Range Achievement
Test

WRC
washed red cells

WRE
whole ragweed extract

ws
water soluble
watt-seconds

WT
wild type

wt
weight

WV
whispered voice

w/v
weight (of solute) per
volume (of solvent)

w/w
weight (of solute) per
weight (of total solution)

X
>cross
>homeopathic symbol for the decimal scale of potencies
>Kienböck's unit
>magnification
>no(t) times
>respirations (anesthesia chart)
>start of anesthesia
>times
>xanthine
>xanthosine

X
>reactance

Xc
>medical decision level

x̄
>except
>mean

x
>abscissa

Ξ
>upper case xi

ξ
>xi, the fourteenth letter of the Greek alphabet

Xan
>xanthine

Xao
>xanthosine

XC
>excretory cystogram

XDP
>xeroderma pigmentosum

Xe
>xenon

XIP
>x-ray in plaster

XLD
>xylose-lysine-deoxycholate (agar)

XM
>crossmatch

XMP
>xanthosine monophosphate

XOAN
>X-linked (Nettleship) ocular albinism

XOP
>x-ray out of plaster

XP
>xeroderma pigmentosum

XR
>x-ray

XRF
>X-ray fluorescence spectrometry

XRG
>Xonics radiography

XRT
>external radiation therapy

XS
>excess
>excessive
>xiphisternum

XT
>exotropia

XU
>excretory urogram

Xu
>x-unit

XX
　normal female
　　chromosome type

XX/XY
　sex karyotypes

XY
　normal male chromosome
　　type

Xyl
　　xylose

Y
yttrium

y
year

y
ordinate

YAC
yeast artificial
chromosome

YAG
yttrium aluminum garnet

Yb
ytterbium

yd
yard

YF
yellow fever

YO
years old

y.o.
years old

YOB
year of birth

YPLL
years of potential life lost

yr
year

YS
yellow spot

Z
> atomic number
> carbobenzoxy
> impedance
> zero
> Ger. Zuckung (contraction)

Z
> atomic number
> impedance

z.
> Z disk

z
> charge

ζ
> zeta, the sixth letter of the Greek alphabet

Z/D
> zero defects

Z-DNA
> a form of DNA

ZDV
> zidovudine

ZE
> Zollinger-Ellison (syndrome)

Z-E
> Zollinger-Ellison syndrome

ZEEP
> zero end-expiratory pressure

ZFY
> zinc finger Y

ZIG
> zoster immune globulin (vaccine)

ZIP
> zoster-immune plasma

Zn
> between
> zinc

Zo_2
> microliters of oxygen taken up per hour by 10^8 spermatozoa

Zr
> zirconium

ZSR
> zeta sedimentation rate

Zz.
> L. zingiber (ginger)

Z.Z.′Z.″
> increasing degrees of contraction

Miscellaneous Symbols

+   acid
         and
         increased
         plus
         positive
         present
         slight trace

++   moderate
         normally active
         noticeable reaction
         trace

+++   increased
         moderately active
         moderately severe

++++ large amount
         pronounced reaction
         severe

++/+   2 plus on the right,
         1 plus on the left

0/0   zero on either side

(+)   significant

−   absent
         alkaline
         decreased
         diminished
         minus
         negative

(−)   insignificant

±   plus or minus
         positive or negative

(±)   possibly significant

×   multiplied by
         times

1×   once

×2   twice

2×   twice

÷   divided by

/   divided by
         of
         per

=   equals

≠   not equal to

≈   approximately equal to

~   approximately

>   greater than
         results in

≯   not greater than

<   less than
         results from

≮   not less than

≥   greater than or
         equal to

≤	less than or equal to
%	percent
°	degree
	hour
1°	first degree
	one hour
	primary
2°	secondary
	second degree
	two hours
3°	tertiary
	third degree
24°	24 hours
′	foot
	minute
	univalent
″	bivalent
	inch
	second
:	is to
	ratio
::	as (in ratios)
∴	therefore
#	fracture
	gauge
	has been done
	has been given
	number
	pounds
@	at
∞	indefinitely more
	infinite
	infinity
Δt	time interval
‖	parallel
	parallel bars

↑	elevated
	gas
	increased
	increasing
↑↑	extensor response, Babinski sign
	testes undescended
↓	decreased
	decreasing
	deficiency
	deficit
	depressed
	diminished
	precipitate
↓↓	bilaterally descended
	both down
	plantar response, Babinski sign
	testes descended
→	reaction proceeds to the right
	results in
	transfer to
	yields
←	is due to
	reaction proceeds to the left
⇆	reversible reaction
?	doubtful
	equivocal
	flicker
	possible
	questionable
	unknown
∟	right lower quadrant
	right angle
⌐	right upper quadrant
⌐	left upper quadrant
⌐	left lower quadrant

∧	diastolic blood pressure	*	birth not verified presumed
∨	systolic blood pressure		
√	check observe for	†	dead death died
⊖	normal		
⊙	start of operation	∋	scruple
⊗	end of operation		
∞	male	℈	dram
♂	male	℥	ounce
♀	female	Ω	ohm